Nutrition for Dementia

Nutrition for Dementia

A Dementia Care Essentials Guide

PETER M. ABRAHAM, BSN, RN

Nutrition for Dementia
A Dementia Care Essentials Guide
Copyright © 2024 Peter M. Abraham, BSN, RN

All rights reserved. No part of this book may be reproduced or transmitted in any manner whatsoever without written permission, except for brief quotations embodied in critical articles and reviews. This book is a work of nonfiction intended for educational purposes only.

This book is a work of non-fiction. The views expressed are solely those of the author and do not necessarily reflect the publisher's opinions, and the publisher hereby disclaims any responsibility for them.

Contact Info: author@2abraham.com

First   Edition: August   2024

DEDICATION

This book and the Dementia Care Essentials series it is part of are dedicated to multiple parties that helped shape my experiences and wisdom in caring for loved ones suffering from various types of dementia. I've worked with loved ones with dementia in long-term care as a registered nurse supervisor and as a hospice case manager. Caregivers and family members provided the most significant insights over the years.

Deborah, the wife of an Alzheimer's hospice at-home patient, provided insight into how the brains of dementia patients can be thought of like an electric clock. Most of the time, the clock is short-circuited and, therefore, not working correctly, but at times, as the clock's hands turn, the short-circuit goes away. For a fleeting time, a day or so, the person appears as if they don't have dementia.

Kathy is one of four daughters of a dementia patient for whom I provided care in a memory care center raised thought-provoking questions about the ethical dilemma of waking loved ones with dementia who want to sleep all the time to feed them vs. just letting them sleep.

Linda, who worked alongside me with a dementia patient, a former registered nurse herself, helped me understand other applications of validation therapy (a set of strategies and techniques that will be discussed in this book), such as rolling with resistance, which included accepting the nickname of "Jack," rather than my desire to be called Peter.

Jed, for whom I cared for his mother at home and then within a memory care center, reminded me of the actual cost that cannot be measured in terms of money of being a family caregiver.

Then there's our family journey, where my mother-in-law developed mixed dementia -- Alzheimer's disease plus vascular dementia – and was being cared for at home by her late husband, and then in a memory care center after he died suddenly.

More family members are involved, each helping me gain wisdom not taught in books. It is to all of these families and caregivers, as well as my late mother-in-law, Loris, and my wife, Laura, to whom this book and the others in this series are dedicated.

Table of Contents

Introduction — 1
Caring for the Caregiver — 2
   The Emotional and Physical Toll — 2
   Recognizing the Signs of Caregiver Burnout — 3
   Understanding the Importance of Self-Care — 6
   Physical Self-Care Strategies — 10
   Emotional and Mental Well-being — 16
   Journaling and Emotional Expression — 18
   Seeking Professional Mental Health Support — 20
   Utilizing Community Resources and Respite Care — 26
   Coping with Grief and Loss — 40
   Finding Meaning in the Caregiving Journey — 42
   Self-Advocacy and Setting Boundaries — 44
   Continuing Education and Skills Development — 46

Planning: Legal and Financial Considerations — 50
   Financial and Legal Considerations — 50
   Understanding Legal Rights and Options — 52
   Medical Power of Attorney: What It Is and Why It Matters — 54
   Financial Power of Attorney: Protecting Assets and Finances — 55
   Living Wills and Advance Directives — 56
   When and How to Have These Conversations — 56
   Finding Legal Assistance for Document Preparation — 57
   Exploring Financial Assistance Programs — 59

Validation Therapy — 62
   Naomi Feil's Validation Therapy — 62
   Other Validation Techniques — 65
   Environmental Modifications — 68
   Practical Strategies for Caregivers — 69

Communication Tips for De-escalating Fear _____ 71

Case Studies and Real-Life Examples _____ 73

Nutrition and Dementia _____ 75

Understanding Eating Challenges in Dementia _____ 75

The Role of Nutrition in Brain Health _____ 78

Essential Vitamins and Minerals for Cognitive Function _____ 78

Supplements and Alternative Nutrition Sources _____ 82

Encouraging Independent Eating and Drinking _____ 86

Understanding and Managing Swallowing Difficulties (Dysphagia) _____ 89

Preventing Complications: Aspiration Pneumonia _____ 93

Assisting with Feeding: A Compassionate Approach _____ 96

Nutrition in Late-Stage Dementia _____ 99

End-of-Life Nutritional Considerations _____ 103

Practical Tips for Caregivers _____ 107

When to Seek Professional Help _____ 110

Preparing for End-of-Life Decisions _____ 113

When to Consider Hospice _____ 115

The importance of timely hospice involvement _____ 116

Signs It May Be Time for Hospice Care _____ 117

The Benefits of Hospice Care for Dementia Patients _____ 120

Respite care for family caregivers _____ 121

Improved quality of life _____ 122

Common Misconceptions About Hospice Care _____ 123

How to Initiate the Hospice Conversation _____ 127

The Hospice Evaluation Process _____ 130

Preparing for Hospice Care _____ 134

Navigating the Emotional Journey _____ 137

Legal and Financial Considerations _____ 141

Conclusion _____ *145*
Resources _____ *147*
Author Bio _____ *148*

Introduction

I know caring for someone with dementia can be challenging, especially talking about nutrition and the concern over mom, dad, et al. is not eating or eating well enough from your point of view. As an experienced nurse who's worked in long-term care and hospice, I've seen firsthand how difficult it can be for families and caregivers.

Taking care of a loved one with dementia is already a big task. They might not even realize they have dementia, which can make things even trickier. It's like they're moving forward in time physically, but mentally and emotionally, and functionally, they're heading back to being entirely dependent, kind of like a newborn.

That's why I wanted to write this book. I hope it'll give you some helpful strategies for treating nutritional concerns for a loved one with dementia. And don't worry—many of these tips will also benefit other aspects of caregiving!

I've set up this book with you in mind. We'll start by discussing why it's so crucial for you to take care of yourself. When someone you love has a serious, long-term illness like dementia (which can last for decades), it affects the whole family. The person with dementia isn't the only one suffering - caregivers like you are going through a lot, too.

After we cover self-care and some practical tips, we will discuss the importance of early legal and financial planning, which is crucial to protect yourself and your loved one. Then, we'll discuss validation therapy and other ways to communicate better with your loved one. Trust me, these skills will come in handy in all sorts of tricky situations, not just with dementia care.

Once we've covered those basics, we'll get into the nitty-gritty of nutrition for loved ones with dementia. Since many people with dementia eventually need end-of-life care, we'll wrap up by covering that vital topic, too.

I'm here to help you through this journey. It isn't easy, but you can do it with the right tools and support. Remember, you're not alone in this!

Caring for the Caregiver

Caring for a loved one with dementia is a journey of profound love and dedication, but it's also one of the most challenging roles a person can undertake. As caregivers and family members, you stand at the forefront of this complex and often overwhelming experience. Your commitment to providing compassionate care is admirable, yet it's crucial to recognize the significant impact this role can have on your well-being.

The Emotional and Physical Toll

The path of a dementia caregiver is paved with a myriad of emotions and physical demands that can test even the strongest individuals. Let's explore the multifaceted nature of this toll:

Emotional Challenges:

1. Grief and loss: Watching a loved one's cognitive decline
2. Guilt: Feeling inadequate or struggling with difficult decisions
3. Anxiety: Worrying about the future and managing daily uncertainties
4. Frustration: Dealing with repetitive behaviors and communication barriers
5. Isolation: Experiencing a shrinking social circle and loss of personal time

Physical Demands:

- Sleep deprivation due to irregular sleep patterns of the care recipient
- Chronic stress leading to weakened immune function
- Neglect of personal health needs and medical appointments
- Physical strain from assisting with mobility and personal care tasks
- Exhaustion from constant vigilance and round-the-clock care

These emotional and physical challenges create a complex web that can entangle even the most resilient caregivers. It's essential to recognize that experiencing these difficulties doesn't reflect on your capabilities or dedication – it's a natural response to an extraordinarily demanding situation.

Common Caregiver Emotions	Physical Manifestations	Potential Long-term Consequences
Sadness, Grief	Fatigue, Weakened Immunity	Depression, Chronic Illness
Anxiety, Worry	Insomnia, Muscle Tension	Anxiety Disorders, Chronic Pain
Frustration, Anger	High Blood Pressure, Headaches	Cardiovascular Issues, Migraines
Guilt, Self-doubt	Appetite Changes, Digestive Issues	Eating Disorders, Gastrointestinal Problems

Recognizing the Signs of Caregiver Burnout

Caregiver burnout is a state of physical, emotional, and mental exhaustion that can creep up slowly or suddenly. Awareness of the warning signs is crucial to prevent reaching this critical point. Here are key indicators to watch for:

1. **Emotional Signs:**
    - Feeling overwhelmed or constantly worried
    - Experiencing mood swings or irritability
    - Losing interest in activities once enjoyed
    - Feeling hopeless, helpless, or alone

2. **Physical Signs:**
    - Frequently falling ill or feeling constantly tired
    - Changes in appetite or sleep patterns
    - Neglecting personal hygiene or appearance
    - Developing new health problems or exacerbating existing ones

3. **Behavioral Signs:**
    - Withdrawing from friends and family
    - Procrastinating on important tasks
    - Using alcohol, food, or medications to cope
    - Lashing out at the person with dementia or others

4. **Cognitive Signs:**
    - Difficulty concentrating or making decisions
    - Forgetfulness in daily tasks
    - Trouble problem-solving or thinking clearly
    - Negative thought patterns or constant worry

Self-Assessment Checklist for Caregiver Burnout:

Warning Sign	Frequency (Rarely/Sometimes/Often/Always)
I feel exhausted even after sleeping.	
I catch myself yelling or arguing more often.	
I've stopped seeing friends or engaging in hobbies.	
I feel resentful towards the person I'm caring for.	
I worry constantly about the future.	
I neglect my own health needs.	
I have trouble falling asleep or staying asleep.	
I feel like I can't do anything right.	

If you find yourself answering "Often" or "Always" to several of these statements, it may be time to seek additional support and focus on self-care strategies.

Remember, recognizing these signs is not an admission of failure but a crucial step in maintaining your ability to provide care. By acknowledging the challenges and being vigilant about your well-being, you can take proactive steps to prevent burnout and ensure that you can continue to provide the best possible care for your loved one with dementia. Your role is invaluable, and by taking care of yourself, you're also ensuring the best care for your loved one.

Understanding the Importance of Self-Care

As caregivers and family members supporting individuals with dementia, you're intimately familiar with the concept of care. However, it's crucial to remember that care must also extend to you. Self-care isn't a luxury; it's a necessity that directly impacts your ability to provide compassionate, practical support to your loved ones or patients.

The Impact of Self-Care on Caregiving Quality

The quality of care you provide is intrinsically linked to your well-being. When you prioritize self-care, you benefit yourself and enhance your capacity to care for others. Let's explore how self-care positively influences various aspects of caregiving:

1. **Enhanced Emotional Resilience**

    - Better equipped to handle stress and emotional challenges
    - Increased patience and empathy in difficult situations
    - Improved ability to maintain a calm demeanor

2. **Improved Physical Stamina**

    - Greater energy to perform caregiving tasks
    - Reduced risk of caregiver-related injuries
    - Increased overall health, leading to fewer sick days

3. **Sharpened Mental Acuity**

    - Better decision-making skills in critical situations
    - Improved memory and attention to detail
    - Enhanced problem-solving abilities

4. **Strengthened Relationships**

    - more positive interactions with the care recipient

- Healthier boundaries with family members and healthcare professionals
- Improved communication skills

5. **Increased Caregiving Longevity**
    - Reduced risk of burnout and compassion fatigue
    - Sustained ability to provide care over extended periods
    - Greater job satisfaction for professional caregivers

Self-Care Practice	Benefits to Caregiver	Impact on Caregiving Quality
Regular Exercise	Improved physical health, stress relief	Increased energy, better mood during care
Adequate Sleep	Better cognitive function, emotional stability	Enhanced decision-making, patience in care
Mindfulness/Meditation	Reduced anxiety, improved focus	Increased presence and empathy in interactions
Social Connections	Emotional support, reduced isolation	Renewed energy and perspective in caregiving

Overcoming Guilt and Prioritizing Personal Needs

One of the most significant barriers to self-care for caregivers is the pervasive feeling of guilt. It's common to feel that taking time for yourself is selfish or detracts from the care you should provide. However, overcoming this guilt is essential for sustainable caregiving. Here's how to reframe your thinking and prioritize your needs:

Understanding Guilt in Caregiving:

- Recognize that guilt is a common and normal emotion for caregivers
- Acknowledge that guilt often stems from unrealistic expectations of yourself
- Realize that neglecting your needs can lead to resentment and diminished care quality

Strategies for Overcoming Caregiver Guilt:

1. **Reframe Your Perspective**
    - View self-care as a necessary part of providing good care
    - Understand that taking care of yourself allows you to be more present and effective
    - Recognize that you're modeling healthy behavior for others

2. **Set Realistic Expectations**
    - Accept that you can't do everything perfectly
    - Understand that it's okay to have limits and boundaries
    - Recognize that asking for help is a sign of strength, not weakness

3. **Practice Self-Compassion**
    - Treat yourself with the same kindness you show to others
    - Acknowledge your efforts and successes, no matter how small
    - Use positive self-talk to counter guilty thoughts

4. **Educate Yourself and Others**
   - Learn about the importance of self-care in caregiving literature
   - Share information with family members to gain their support
   - Discuss the benefits of caregiver well-being with healthcare professionals

5. **Start Small and Build**
   - Begin with short periods of self-care to ease into the practice
   - Gradually increase the time and frequency of self-care activities
   - Celebrate each step you take towards prioritizing your needs

Practical Steps to Prioritize Personal Needs:

- **Schedule Self-Care**: Block out time in your calendar for activities that rejuvenate you
- **Create a Self-Care Plan**: Develop a written plan outlining your self-care goals and strategies
- **Communicate Your Needs**: Clearly express your needs to family members and support networks
- **Use Respite Care**: Take advantage of respite services to get regular breaks
- **Join Support Groups**: Connect with other caregivers who understand your challenges
- **Seek Professional Help**: Consider therapy or counseling to work through feelings of guilt

Common Guilt-Inducing Thoughts	Reframed Perspective
"I should be doing more."	"I'm doing my best, and that's enough."
"Taking a break is selfish."	"Taking care of myself helps me provide better care."
"Nobody else can care for them like I can."	"Accepting help allows for fresh energy in caregiving."
"I don't deserve to enjoy myself."	"My well-being is important and valid."

Remember, prioritizing your needs isn't selfish—it's essential. You can continue providing the high-quality, compassionate care that your loved ones or patients deserve by taking care of yourself. Self-care is integral to the caregiving journey, benefiting you and those you care for. Embrace it without guilt, knowing that you're making a wise investment in your ability to care for others.

Physical Self-Care Strategies

Your physical health is the foundation of your ability to provide care as a caregiver. While putting your needs last is easy, maintaining your physical well-being is crucial for you and your loved one. Let's explore practical strategies to keep your body healthy and energized.

Maintaining a Healthy Diet

A nutritious diet is essential for sustaining your energy levels and overall health. Here are some strategies to ensure you're fueling your body properly:

1. **Plan and Prepare Meals in Advance**
   - Use weekends or less busy times to batch-cook meals
   - Freeze portions for easy reheating during hectic days
   - Prepare healthy snacks to avoid reaching for processed foods

2. **Focus on Nutrient-Dense Foods**

- Incorporate a variety of colorful fruits and vegetables
- Choose whole grains over refined carbohydrates
- Include lean proteins like fish, poultry, beans, and nuts
- Don't forget healthy fats from sources like avocados and olive oil

3. **Stay Hydrated**
   - Keep a water bottle with you throughout the day
   - Set reminders to drink water regularly
   - Include hydrating foods like cucumbers and watermelon in your diet

4. **Mindful Eating**
   - Take time to sit down and enjoy your meals
   - Avoid eating while multitasking or when stressed
   - Listen to your body's hunger and fullness cues

5. **Seek Support**
   - Ask family members or friends to help with meal preparation
   - Consider meal delivery services for fresh, healthy options
   - Consult a nutritionist for personalized dietary advice if needed

Meal Type	Quick and Healthy Options
Breakfast	Greek yogurt with berries and nuts, overnight oats, whole grain toast with avocado.
Lunch	Mixed green salad with grilled chicken, whole grain wrap with hummus and vegetables.
Dinner	Baked salmon with roasted vegetables, vegetarian chili, stir-fry with tofu and mixed veggies.
Snacks	Apple slices with almond butter, carrot sticks with hummus, and a handful of mixed nuts.

Incorporating Regular Exercise

Exercise is not just about physical fitness; it's a powerful stress reliever and mood booster. Here's how to make physical activity a regular part of your routine:

1. **Find Activities You Enjoy**
   - Experiment with different types of exercise to find what you like
   - Consider activities that can involve your loved one, like gentle walks
   - Try yoga or tai chi for both physical and mental benefits

2. **Set Realistic Goals**
   - Start small. Even 10 minutes a day can make a difference
   - Gradually increase duration and intensity as you build stamina
   - Celebrate your progress, no matter how small

3. **Make It Convenient**
    - Keep exercise equipment at home for quick workouts
    - Use online fitness videos for guided sessions
    - Take advantage of small pockets of time throughout the day

4. **Incorporate Movement into Daily Tasks**
    - Do calf raises while washing dishes
    - Perform stretches during TV commercials
    - Take the stairs instead of the elevator when possible

5. **Seek Support and Accountability**
    - Join a caregiver fitness group or online community
    - Use fitness apps to track your progress
    - Ask a friend or family member to be your exercise buddy

Exercise Type	Benefits	Caregiver-Friendly Examples
Cardiovascular	Improves heart health, boosts energy	Brisk walking, dancing, stationary cycling
Strength Training	Builds muscle, supports bone health	Bodyweight exercises, resistance bands, light dumbbells
Flexibility	Reduces muscle tension, improves mobility	Gentle stretching, yoga, tai chi
Balance	Prevents falls, improves stability	Single-leg stands, heel-to-toe walk, balance board

Ensuring Adequate Sleep and Rest

Quality sleep is crucial for your physical and mental well-being. Here are strategies to improve your sleep habits:

1. **Establish a Consistent Sleep Schedule**
    - Try to go to bed and wake up at the same time each day
    - Create a relaxing bedtime routine to signal your body it's time to sleep
    - Avoid screens for at least an hour before bedtime

2. **Optimize Your Sleep Environment**
    - Keep your bedroom cool, dark, and quiet
    - Invest in a comfortable mattress and pillows
    - Use white noise or earplugs if needed to block out disturbances

3. **Manage Nighttime Caregiving**
    - Use night lights to avoid fully waking up for nighttime checks
    - Consider assistive devices like bed alarms to alert you when needed
    - Take turns with other family members for nighttime care if possible

4. **Practice Relaxation Techniques**
    - Try deep breathing exercises before bed
    - Use guided imagery or meditation to calm your mind
    - Practice progressive muscle relaxation to release physical tension

5. **Be Mindful of Diet and Exercise**
    - Avoid caffeine and heavy meals close to bedtime
    - Exercise regularly, but not too close to bedtime
    - Limit alcohol, as it can disrupt sleep patterns

6. **Prioritize Rest During the Day**
    - Take short power naps (15-20 minutes) when possible
    - Use respite care to get a whole night's sleep occasionally
    - Practice mindfulness or meditation for mental rest during the day

Sleep Challenge	Potential Solution
Difficulty falling asleep	Practice a calming bedtime routine, and try relaxation techniques.
Waking up during the night	Keep a notepad by your bed to jot down thoughts, and use white noise.
Early morning wakings	Ensure your room is dark, and consider adjusting your sleep schedule.
Feeling unrested after sleep	Evaluate your sleep environment and consult a doctor about sleep quality.

Remember, taking care of your physical health is not selfish—it's a necessary part of being an effective caregiver. By prioritizing your diet, exercise, and sleep, you're ensuring you have the strength and energy to provide the best care possible for your loved one. Start with small, manageable changes, and be patient with yourself as you develop these healthy habits. Your body—and your loved one—will thank you for it.

Emotional and Mental Well-being

As a caregiver, tending to your emotional and mental health is just as crucial as maintaining your physical well-being. The demands of caring for a loved one can significantly toll your psychological state, making it essential to develop strategies that nurture your inner self. Let's explore some effective methods to support your emotional and mental well-being.

Practicing Mindfulness and Meditation

Mindfulness and meditation are powerful tools for managing stress, improving focus, and cultivating inner peace. These practices can be particularly beneficial for caregivers, offering moments of calm in challenging situations.

Benefits of Mindfulness and Meditation for Caregivers:

- Reduced stress and anxiety
- Improved emotional regulation
- Enhanced ability to focus and concentrate
- Increased self-awareness and empathy
- Better sleep quality
- Boosted immune function

How to Incorporate Mindfulness and Meditation into Your Daily Routine:

1. **Start Small**
    - Begin with just 5 minutes a day
    - Gradually increase the duration as you become more comfortable

2. **Choose a Consistent Time and Place**
    - Set aside a specific time each day for your practice
    - Create a quiet, comfortable space for meditation

3. **Explore Different Techniques**
   - Try guided meditations using apps or online resources
   - Experiment with breathing exercises, body scans, or loving-kindness meditation
   - Practice mindful activities like walking or eating

4. **Be Patient and Non-Judgmental**
   - Remember that it's normal for your mind to wander
   - Gently bring your attention back to your focus point without self-criticism

5. **Integrate Mindfulness into Daily Activities**
   - Practice being fully present during routine tasks like washing dishes or folding laundry
   - Take mindful breaks throughout the day, even if just for a few deep breaths

Mindfulness Technique	Description	When to Use
Breath Awareness	Focus on the sensation of breathing, noticing each inhale and exhale	Any time, especially during stressful moments
Body Scan	Systematically relax each part of your body from head to toe	Before bed or during breaks
Loving-Kindness Meditation	Direct positive thoughts and wishes towards yourself and others	When feeling overwhelmed or frustrated
Mindful Walking	Pay attention to each step and your surroundings while walking	During outdoor breaks or while moving between tasks

Journaling and Emotional Expression

Journaling is a powerful tool for processing emotions, gaining clarity, and fostering self-reflection. For caregivers, it can serve as a private outlet for expressing the complex feelings often accompanying caregiving.

Benefits of Journaling for Caregivers:

- Emotional release and stress reduction
- Increased self-awareness and problem-solving
- Documentation of caregiving journey and memories
- Opportunity for a gratitude practice
- Improved communication skills

Tips for Effective Journaling:

1. **Choose Your Medium**
   - Traditional pen and paper
   - Digital journaling apps or word processors
   - Audio recordings or voice memos

2. **Set Aside Regular Time**
   - Aim for consistency, even if it's just a few minutes daily
   - Choose a time when you're least likely to be interrupted

3. **Write Freely Without Judgment**
   - Don't worry about grammar, spelling, or structure
   - Let your thoughts flow without censoring yourself

4. **Use Prompts When Needed**
    - "Today, I felt..."
    - "I'm grateful for..."
    - "A challenge I faced today was..."
    - "Something I learned about myself is..."

5. **Reflect on Your Entries**
    - Periodically review your journal to observe patterns and growth
    - Use insights gained to inform your self-care and caregiving strategies

6. **Explore Different Journaling Techniques**
    - Gratitude journaling
    - Stream of consciousness writing
    - Dialogue journaling (writing conversations with yourself or others)
    - Art journaling (combining writing with visual elements)

Journaling Method	Description	Benefit for Caregivers
Gratitude Journal	Daily list of things you're thankful for	Shifts focus to positive aspects of caregiving
Emotional Release Writing	Unfiltered expression of feelings and thoughts	Helps process difficult emotions and experiences
Problem-Solving Journal	Writing out challenges and brainstorming solutions	Enhances coping skills and decision-making
Reflection Journal	Regular entries about personal growth and insights	Promotes self-awareness and resilience

Seeking Professional Mental Health Support

While self-care practices are essential, there may be times when professional support is necessary. Seeking help from a mental health professional is a sign of strength and can provide valuable tools for managing the emotional challenges of caregiving.

Signs You May Benefit from Professional Support:

- Persistent feelings of sadness, anxiety, or hopelessness
- Difficulty managing anger or frustration
- Feeling overwhelmed or unable to cope
- Changes in sleep patterns or appetite
- Loss of interest in activities you once enjoyed
- Thoughts of self-harm or suicide

Types of Professional Mental Health Support:

1. **Individual Therapy**
    - One-on-one sessions with a licensed therapist or counselor.
    - Can focus on specific caregiving challenges or broader emotional issues.

2. **Support Groups**
    - Facilitated groups for caregivers to share experiences and coping strategies.
    - It can be in-person or online.

3. **Cognitive Behavioral Therapy (CBT)**
    - It helps identify and change negative thought patterns and behaviors.
    - It is particularly effective for managing anxiety and depression.

4. **Mindfulness-Based Stress Reduction (MBSR)**
   - Combines mindfulness meditation and yoga to reduce stress.
   - Often offered in 8-week programs.

5. **Telehealth Options**
   - Virtual therapy sessions via video call or phone.
   - Convenient for caregivers with limited time or transportation.

Steps to Access Mental Health Support:

1. **Consult Your Primary Care Physician**
   - Discuss your concerns and get referrals to mental health professionals.

2. **Check with Your Insurance Provider**
   - Understand your coverage for mental health services.
   - Get a list of in-network providers.

3. **Research Local Resources**
   - Contact local hospitals or community centers for caregiver support programs.
   - Look into non-profit organizations specializing in your loved one's condition.

4. **Consider Online Platforms**
   - Explore reputable online therapy services.
   - Look for platforms that offer specific support for caregivers.

5. **Don't Hesitate to Try Different Options**
    - Switching therapists is okay if you don't feel a good connection.
    - Explore different types of therapy to find what works best for you.

Type of Support	Best For	Potential Drawbacks
Individual Therapy	Personalized attention, deep exploration of issues	It can be costly, time-consuming
Support Groups	Shared experiences, practical advice from peers	Less individual focus and may not address specific needs
Online Therapy	Convenience, flexibility in scheduling	Potential technology issues, less personal connection
Crisis Hotlines	Immediate support during acute stress or emergencies	Not suitable for ongoing, in-depth support

Remember, taking care of your emotional and mental well-being is not a luxury—it's a necessity. By practicing mindfulness, journaling, and seeking professional support when needed, you're investing in your ability to provide compassionate care. Be patient with yourself as you explore these strategies, and remember that it's okay to prioritize your mental health. A mentally healthy caregiver is better equipped to face the challenges of caregiving with resilience and grace.

Building a Support Network

As a caregiver, it's crucial to remember that you don't have to face this journey alone. Building a solid support network can provide emotional support, practical assistance, and valuable resources. Let's explore how you can create and nurture a network that will sustain you through the challenges of caregiving.

Joining Caregiver Support Groups

Caregiver support groups offer a unique opportunity to connect with others who truly understand your experiences. These groups can be invaluable sources of emotional support, practical advice, and camaraderie.

Benefits of Joining Caregiver Support Groups:

- Emotional validation and understanding
- Sharing of practical tips and resources
- Reduced feelings of isolation and loneliness
- Opportunity to help others and feel empowered
- Access to educational resources and expert speakers

Types of Caregiver Support Groups:

1. **In-Person Groups**
    - Often held at community centers, hospitals, or religious organizations
    - Provide face-to-face interaction and immediate support

2. **Online Forums and Groups**
    - Accessible from anywhere, at any time
    - Offer anonymity and convenience

3. **Condition-Specific Groups**
    - Focus on caregivers dealing with particular illnesses or conditions
    - Provide specialized information and understanding

4. **Demographic-Specific Groups**
    - Cater to specific caregiver demographics (e.g., spouses, adult children, young caregivers)
    - Address unique challenges faced by different caregiver populations

How to Find and Join a Support Group:

1. Research local options through hospitals, community centers, or disease-specific organizations
2. Explore online platforms like Facebook groups or caregiver-specific websites
3. Ask your healthcare provider for recommendations
4. Consider starting your group if you can't find one that meets your needs

Type of Group	Pros	Cons
In-Person	Personal connection, immediate support	Time commitment, transportation needed
Online	Convenient, accessible 24/7	Lack of face-to-face interaction
Condition-Specific	Targeted advice, shared experiences	It may be limited in availability
General Caregiver	Broader perspective, diverse experiences	May lack specificity for your situation

Involving Family and Friends

Your existing network of family and friends can be a powerful source of support. However, many caregivers struggle with asking for help or feel guilty about burdening others. Remember, most people want to help but may not know how.

Strategies for Involving Family and Friends:

1. **Be Specific About Your Needs**
   - Create a list of tasks that others can help with
   - Be clear about what kind of support you're looking for (practical, emotional, etc.)

2. **Use Technology to Coordinate**
    - Utilize care coordination apps or shared calendars
    - Set up a group chat or email thread for updates and requests

3. **Educate Them About Your Caregiving Situation**
    - Share information about your loved one's condition
    - Help them understand the challenges you face

4. **Foster Ongoing Connections**
    - Schedule regular check-ins or social gatherings
    - Encourage friends and family to maintain a relationship with your care recipient

5. **Express Gratitude**
    - Thank helpers for their support, no matter how small
    - Let them know the positive impact of their assistance

Overcoming Barriers to Asking for Help:

- Recognize that accepting help benefits both you and your care recipient
- Start small if you're uncomfortable asking for big favors
- Remember that people often want to help but don't know how

Practice asking for help to become more comfortable with it Type of Support	Examples	How to Ask
Practical Assistance	Meal preparation, house cleaning, errands	"Could you pick up groceries for us this week?"
Respite Care	Sitting with the care recipient, overnight care	"Can you stay with Mom for a few hours on Saturday?"
Emotional Support	Listening, checking in, offering encouragement	"I'm having a tough week. Could we chat over coffee?"
Financial Help	Assistance with bills, fundraising	"We're struggling with medical expenses. Can you help us set up a fundraiser?"

Utilizing Community Resources and Respite Care

Community resources and respite care services can provide crucial support, allowing you to take breaks and access specialized assistance. These resources can help prevent burnout and ensure better care for you and your loved one.

Types of Community Resources:

1. **Area Agencies on Aging (AAA)**
    - Provide information, referrals, and sometimes direct services
    - Often offer caregiver support programs and resources

2. **Local Senior Centers**
    - o May offer adult daycare programs
    - o Provide social activities and meals for seniors
3. **Faith-Based Organizations**
    - o Often have volunteer programs to assist caregivers
    - o May offer support groups or counseling services
4. **Non-Profit Organizations**
    - o Condition-specific organizations often have local chapters with resources
    - o May offer educational workshops, support groups, or financial assistance

Respite Care Options:

1. **In-Home Respite**
    - o Professional caregivers come to your home
    - o Can range from a few hours to overnight care
2. **Adult Day Centers**
    - o Provide care and activities during daytime hours
    - o Often include meals and social interaction for care recipients
3. **Residential Respite**
    - o Short-term stays at assisted living facilities or nursing homes
    - o Allows for extended breaks or travel
4. **Volunteer Respite Programs**
    - o Often run by community organizations or faith groups
    - o May offer limited hours of free care

Steps to Access Community Resources and Respite Care:

1. Contact your local AAA for a comprehensive list of resources
2. Speak with your loved one's healthcare provider for recommendations
3. Research condition-specific organizations for specialized support
4. Explore online directories of senior services and respite care options
5. Consult with a social worker or case manager for personalized guidance

Resource Type	Services Offered	How to Access
Area Agency on Aging	Information, referrals, caregiver support programs	Call the local office or visit the website
Adult Day Centers	Daytime care, activities, meals	Contact the center directly for a tour and assessment
Home Health Agencies	In-home care, nursing services, respite	Get a referral from a doctor or contact an agency
Volunteer Programs	Companionship, errands, light housekeeping	Contact local senior centers or faith organizations

Remember, building a strong support network is an ongoing process. Finding the right combination of support groups, family involvement, and community resources that work for you may take time. Be patient with yourself and persistent in seeking out the help you need. By creating a robust support system, you're taking care of yourself and ensuring you can provide the best possible care for your loved one.

Don't hesitate to reach out and accept help when it's offered. Your role as a caregiver is invaluable, and by taking care of yourself through building a strong support network, you're ensuring that you can continue to provide compassionate care for the long term.

Time Management and Organization

As a caregiver, you often juggle multiple responsibilities, making time management and organization crucial skills. Effective planning can help reduce stress, increase efficiency, and ensure you and your loved one receive the care and attention needed. Let's explore strategies to help you manage your time and effectively organize your caregiving duties.

Creating a Caregiving Schedule

A well-structured caregiving schedule can provide a sense of routine and predictability, which benefits both you and your care recipient. Here's how to create an effective caregiving schedule:

1. **Assess Care Needs**
    - List all daily, weekly, and monthly tasks required for your loved one's care.
    - Include medical appointments, medication times, and personal care routines.

2. **Prioritize Tasks**
    - Identify critical tasks that must be done at specific times.
    - Determine which tasks are flexible and can be rescheduled if needed.

3. **Create a Template**
    - Use a digital calendar or a large paper calendar.
    - Color-code different types of activities for easy visualization.

4. **Include Self-Care**
    - Schedule time for your appointments, breaks, and activities.
    - Block out time for sleep and regular meals.

5. **Be Realistic**
    - Allow extra time for tasks, as caregiving often takes longer than expected.
    - Build buffer time for unexpected events or emergencies.
6. **Review and Adjust Regularly**
    - Reassess the schedule weekly or monthly.
    - Make changes as care needs evolve or your situation changes.

Time	Task	Responsible Person
7:00 AM	Morning medications and breakfast	Primary Caregiver
9:00 AM	Personal care and dressing	Home Health Aide
11:00 AM	Physical therapy exercises	Primary Caregiver
1:00 PM	Lunch and afternoon medications	Family Member
3:00 PM	Social activity or rest	Volunteer Companion
6:00 PM	Dinner and evening medications	Primary Caregiver
8:00 PM	Bedtime routine	Primary Caregiver

Delegating Tasks and Accepting Help

Delegating tasks and accepting help are essential for maintaining your well-being and ensuring comprehensive care for your loved one. Here's how to approach delegation effectively:

1. **Identify Delegable Tasks**
    - Make a list of tasks that don't require your specific expertise.
    - Consider which tasks others might enjoy or be well-suited to perform.

2. **Match Tasks to Helpers**
    - Consider the skills, availability, and preferences of potential helpers.
    - Assign tasks that align with each person's strengths and schedules.

3. **Communicate Clearly**
    - Provide detailed instructions for each task.
    - Set clear expectations for how and when tasks should be completed.

4. **Express Appreciation**
    - Thank helpers for their contributions, no matter how small.
    - Acknowledge the positive impact of their assistance.

5. **Be Open to Different Methods**
    - Recognize that others may complete tasks differently than you would.
    - Focus on results rather than specific methods when possible.

6. **Overcome Reluctance to Delegate**
    - Remind yourself that accepting help benefits both you and your loved one.
    - Start small if you're uncomfortable with extensive delegation.

Strategies for Effective Delegation:
- Use a shared task list or care coordination app.
- Rotate responsibilities among family members.
- Consider hiring professional help for specialized tasks.
- Utilize volunteer services for non-medical assistance.

Task Category	Examples	Potential Delegates
Household Chores	Cleaning, laundry, yard work	Family members, hired help, volunteers
Errands	Grocery shopping, pharmacy runs	Friends, neighbors, delivery services
Personal Care	Bathing, dressing, grooming	Home health aides, trained family members
Social Support	Companionship, activities	Friends, volunteers, adult day programs
Medical Management	Medication reminders, doctor appointments	Nursing services, tech solutions, family members

Using Technology to Streamline Caregiving Duties

Technology can be a powerful ally in managing caregiving responsibilities. Various tools can help simplify your caregiving journey, from organizing tasks to monitoring health. Here's how to leverage technology effectively:

1. **Care Coordination Apps**

    o Use apps designed for caregivers to manage schedules, tasks, and communication.

    o Examples: Caring Village, Lotsa Helping Hands, and CaringBridge.

2. **Medication Management Tools**

    o Utilize apps or smart pill dispensers to track and remind about medications.

    o Consider: Medisafe, PillPack, and Hero.

3. **Health Monitoring Devices**
    - Implement wearable devices or smart home sensors for health tracking.
    - Options: Fall detection devices, blood pressure monitors, GPS trackers.

4. **Communication Tools**
    - Use video calling apps to connect with your loved one and other caregivers.
    - Try: Skype, FaceTime, or Zoom.

5. **Online Support and Education**
    - Access online forums, webinars, and caregiver support and education courses.
    - Explore: Family Caregiver Alliance, AARP Caregiver Resource Center.

6. **Smart Home Devices**
    - Implement voice-activated assistants and smart home technology for added convenience and safety.
    - Consider: Amazon Alexa, Google Home, smart thermostats, and automated lighting.

Tips for Implementing Caregiving Technology:

- Start with one or two tools and gradually add more as needed.
- Ensure all caregivers are trained on how to use the technology.
- Regularly review and update your tech tools as care needs change.
- Consider the comfort level of your care recipient with technology.

Technology Type	Benefits	Considerations
Care Coordination Apps	Improved communication, task management	Requires all caregivers to adopt and use consistently
Health Monitoring Devices	Early detection of health issues, increased independence	It may require professional setup, ongoing costs
Medication Management Tools	Reduced medication errors, improved adherence	Need for regular updates, potential tech glitches
Smart Home Devices	Enhanced safety, convenience for daily tasks	Initial setup cost, learning curve for usage

Remember, effective time management and organization are ongoing processes. Be patient with yourself as you implement these strategies, and don't hesitate to adjust your approach as needed. You can create a more manageable and sustainable caregiving routine by creating a structured schedule, delegating tasks, and leveraging technology.

These tools and strategies are meant to support you, not add stress. Please choose the best methods for your unique situation and gradually incorporate them into your caregiving routine. With time and practice, you'll likely find that improved organization leads to more quality time with your loved one and better self-care for you as a caregiver.

Maintaining Personal Identity and Interests

As a caregiver, it's easy to become so immersed in your responsibilities that you lose sight of your identity and interests. However, maintaining a sense of self is crucial for your well-being and can make you a more effective caregiver. Let's explore ways to nurture your identity and interests while balancing your caregiving duties.

Pursuing Hobbies and Passions

Engaging in activities you enjoy is not a luxury—it's necessary to maintain your mental and emotional health. Here's how to keep your hobbies and passions alive:

1. **Identify Time Pockets**
   - Look for small windows of time in your schedule
   - Consider early mornings, during care recipient's naps, or after bedtime

2. **Adapt Your Hobbies**
   - Find ways to engage in your interests in shorter time frames
   - Look for portable versions of your hobbies

3. **Involve Your Care Recipient**
   - When possible, find ways to include your loved one in your activities
   - This can provide stimulation for them and enjoyment for you both

4. **Use Technology**
   - Explore online classes or virtual communities related to your interests
   - Use apps or online resources to engage in hobbies remotely

5. **Schedule Regular "Me Time"**
   - Block out time in your calendar for your interests
   - Treat this time as crucial as any other appointment

Ideas for Maintaining Hobbies:

- Reading: Join an online book club or use audiobooks during commutes
- Art: Keep a sketchbook for quick drawing sessions
- Music: Create playlists to enjoy while performing caregiving tasks
- Gardening: Start a small indoor herb garden or tend to potted plants
- Exercise: Try short workout videos or practice yoga during breaks

Hobby Type	Adaptation for Caregivers	Benefits
Reading	E-books, audiobooks, short stories	Mental stimulation, stress relief
Crafting	Portable projects (knitting, sketching)	Creativity outlet, sense of accomplishment
Fitness	Short home workouts, walking	Physical health, energy boost
Cooking	Quick recipes, meal prep	Nutrition, enjoyment, potential involvement of care recipient

Staying Connected with Friends

Maintaining social connections is vital for your emotional well-being and provides a support system outside your caregiving role. Here are strategies to stay connected:

1. **Leverage Technology**

    - Use video calls, social media, or messaging apps to stay in touch
    - Join online groups or forums related to your interests

2. **Schedule Regular Check-ins**
    - Set up recurring phone calls or virtual coffee dates with friends
    - Use calendar reminders to prompt you to reach out
3. **Be Honest About Your Situation**
    - Share your caregiving challenges with trusted friends
    - Let them know how they can support you
4. **Plan for Social Activities**
    - Arrange respite care to allow for occasional outings
    - Invite friends for short visits at home when possible
5. **Involve Friends in Caregiving**
    - Ask friends to visit or spend time with your care recipient
    - This can provide you with a break while maintaining connections

Tips for Maintaining Friendships:

- Quality over quantity: Focus on nurturing a few close relationships
- Be present: When you do have time with friends, try to be fully engaged
- Share your caregiving journey: Allow friends to understand your life
- Accept help: Let friends support you in practical ways if they offer

Connection Type	Ideas for Caregivers	Potential Challenges
Virtual Meetups	Video chat coffee dates, online game nights	Technology issues, scheduling conflicts
In-Person Visits	Short home visits, park meetups	Limited time, need for care coverage
Group Activities	Book clubs, virtual workout groups	Finding common interests, time commitment
Caregiving Involvement	Friend visits with care recipient, help with tasks	Friends' comfort level with caregiving situation

Setting Personal Goals Outside of Caregiving

Setting and working towards personal goals can provide a sense of purpose and achievement beyond your caregiving role. Here's how to approach goal-setting:

1. **Reflect on Your Aspirations**
   - Think about what you want to achieve for yourself
   - Consider short-term and long-term goals
2. **Start Small**
   - Set realistic, achievable goals given your current situation
   - Break larger goals into smaller, manageable steps
3. **Make Goals SMART**
   - Specific, Measurable, Achievable, Relevant, Time-bound
   - This framework helps create clear, actionable goals

4. **Write Down Your Goals**
    - Use a journal or goal-tracking app to document your objectives
    - Regularly review and update your goals

5. **Seek Support**
    - Share your goals with friends or family who can encourage you
    - Consider finding an accountability partner

6. **Celebrate Progress**
    - Acknowledge and celebrate each step towards your goals
    - Use achievements as motivation to continue pursuing your aspirations

Examples of Personal Goals for Caregivers:

- Learning: Take an online course or learn a new language
- Health: Establish a regular exercise routine or improve eating habits
- Career: Maintain professional skills or explore part-time work options
- Creative: Start a blog, write a book, or create art
- Personal Growth: Practice mindfulness or develop a new skill

Goal Category	Example Goal	Potential Steps
Education	Complete an online certificate program	Research programs, allocate study time, set completion date
Health and Wellness	Establish a regular meditation practice.	Download the app, start with 5 minutes daily, and gradually increase the time.
Personal Development	Improve time management skills.	Read productivity books, try a time-blocking technique, and use organization apps.
Creative Expression	Write and publish a short story	Set writing schedule, join writing group, research publishing options

Remember, maintaining your identity and interests is not selfish—it's essential for your well-being and can make you a more effective and compassionate caregiver. By pursuing your hobbies, staying connected with friends, and setting personal goals, you're taking care of yourself and bringing fresh energy and perspective to your caregiving role.

Feeling guilty about taking time for yourself is normal, but remember that self-care is crucial to sustainable caregiving—your loved one benefits when you're refreshed, fulfilled, and connected to your identity. Be patient with yourself as you navigate this balance, and don't hesitate to adjust your approach as your caregiving situation evolves. Your growth and well-being are important to you and those you care for.

Coping with Grief and Loss

As a caregiver, you may find yourself navigating complex emotions, including grief and loss, long before your loved one's passing. Understanding and addressing these feelings is crucial for your emotional well-being and ability to provide compassionate care. Let's explore how to cope with these challenging aspects of the caregiving journey.

Acknowledging Anticipatory Grief

Anticipatory grief is the grief experienced before an impending loss. For caregivers, this can begin when a loved one is diagnosed with a progressive illness or when you start to notice significant declines. Recognizing and addressing this grief is an integral part of your emotional health.

Signs of Anticipatory Grief:

- Sadness or tearfulness
- Anxiety about the future
- Loneliness or isolation
- Anger or irritability
- Guilt or regret
- Physical symptoms like fatigue or changes in appetite

Strategies for Coping with Anticipatory Grief:

1. **Acknowledge Your Feelings**
    - Recognize that your grief is valid and normal
    - Allow yourself to experience and express your emotions

2. **Seek Support**
    - Join a caregiver support group
    - Consider talking to a therapist or counselor
    - Confide in trusted friends or family members

3. **Practice Self-Care**
    - Engage in activities that bring you comfort
    - Maintain your physical health through diet and exercise
    - Set aside time for relaxation and stress relief

4. **Create Meaningful Moments**
    - Make new memories with your loved one
    - Document your journey through journaling or photography
    - Engage in life review conversations with your loved one
5. **Educate Yourself**
    - Learn about your loved one's condition and what to expect
    - Understand the grief process and its various manifestations

Emotion	Coping Strategy	Self-Care Action
Sadness	Allow yourself to cry; express emotions through art or writing	Practice gratitude journaling; spend time in nature
Anxiety	Use relaxation techniques; focus on the present moment	Try meditation or deep breathing exercises
Guilt	Challenge negative thoughts; practice self-compassion	Engage in positive self-talk; seek validation from support group
Anger	Find healthy outlets like exercise; communicate feelings assertively	Practice stress-relief techniques; consider counseling

Finding Meaning in the Caregiving Journey

While caregiving can be challenging, many find it offers opportunities for personal growth, deepened relationships, and a sense of purpose. Finding meaning in your caregiving role can help you cope with the difficulties and find moments of joy and fulfillment.

Ways to Find Meaning In Caregiving:

1. **Reflect on Your Values**
   - Consider how caregiving aligns with your values
   - Recognize the positive impact you're making in your loved one's life

2. **Practice Mindfulness**
   - Stay present in the moment, appreciating small joys
   - Use mindfulness techniques to manage stress and find peace

3. **Cultivate Gratitude**
   - Keep a gratitude journal, noting the positive aspects of each day
   - Share moments of appreciation with your loved one

4. **Learn and Grow**
   - View challenges as opportunities for personal development
   - Acquire new skills and knowledge through your caregiving role

5. **Connect with Others**
   - Share your experiences with other caregivers
   - Offer support and mentorship to those new to caregiving

6. **Create a Legacy Project**
   - Work with your loved one to create something meaningful (e.g., a memory book, video, or family history project)

Find ways to honor your loved one's life and values Aspect of Caregiving	Potential for Meaning	Action to Cultivate Meaning
Daily Care Tasks	Expressing love through service	Practice mindfulness during care routines
Emotional Support	Deepening relationship bonds	Engage in life review conversations
Learning New Skills	Personal growth and empowerment	Recognize and celebrate your growing expertise
Advocating for Loved One	Standing up for what's right	Reflect on how advocacy aligns with your values

Self-Advocacy and Setting Boundaries

As a caregiver for someone with dementia, you're often so focused on your loved one's needs that you might forget to advocate for yourself. Remember, your well-being is just as important. Let's explore how you can effectively communicate your needs, set boundaries, and maintain a healthy balance in your life.

Communicating needs effectively

Effective communication is critical to meeting your needs while caring for someone with dementia. Here are some strategies to help you communicate more effectively:

1. Be clear and specific about your needs
2. Use "I" statements to express your feelings
3. Choose the right time and place for meaningful conversations
4. Practice active listening when others are speaking
5. Be open to compromise and negotiation

Communication Do's	Communication Don'ts
Express yourself calmly and respectfully.	Use accusatory language or blame others.
Be specific about what you need.	Assume others know what you're thinking.
Listen to others' perspectives.	Interrupt or dismiss others' opinions.
Take time to collect your thoughts.	React impulsively when emotions are high.

Learning to say 'no' when necessary

As a caregiver, you may feel obligated to say 'yes' to every request or task related to your loved one's care. However, learning to say 'no' when necessary is crucial for your well-being and the quality of care you provide. Here's how you can start setting limits:

- Recognize your limits: Be honest about what you can realistically handle.
- Prioritize tasks: Focus on the most essential and remove less critical responsibilities.
- Practice saying 'no': Start small and work up to more significant boundaries.
- Offer alternatives: Suggest other solutions or resources if you can't do something.
- Don't feel guilty: Remember that setting boundaries is healthy and necessary.

Balancing caregiving with other responsibilities

Striking a balance between caregiving and other aspects of your life can be challenging, but it's essential for your overall well-being. Here are some strategies to help you maintain equilibrium:

1. Create a schedule: Allocate time for caregiving, work, family, and personal activities.

2. Delegate tasks: Involve other family members or hire help for specific responsibilities.

3. Use respite care: Take advantage of short-term care options to give yourself a break.

4. Maintain your health: Prioritize your physical and mental well-being through regular check-ups and self-care.

5. Stay connected: Nurture relationships outside of your caregiving role.

Area of Life	Strategies for Balance
Work	Discuss flexible options with your employer, and consider part-time work if possible.
Family	Schedule regular family time and involve children in age-appropriate caregiving tasks.
Personal Time	Set aside time each day for activities you enjoy, even if it's just for 15 minutes.
Social Life	Join a support group and plan regular outings with friends.

Remember, caring for yourself isn't selfish—it's necessary. By advocating for your needs, setting boundaries, and maintaining balance in your life, you'll be better equipped to provide quality care for your loved one with dementia. Don't hesitate to seek support when you need it, whether from family, friends, or professional resources. You're doing important and challenging work and deserve care and support.

Continuing Education and Skills Development

As a caregiver for someone with dementia, your journey is one of continuous learning and growth. Staying informed about the latest care techniques and developing your skills can significantly improve your loved one's quality of life and your caregiving experience. Let's explore how you can enhance your knowledge and abilities in this challenging but rewarding role.

Staying informed about dementia care techniques

Dementia care is an evolving field, with new research and techniques emerging regularly. Keeping up-to-date with these developments can help you provide the best possible care for your loved one. Here are some ways to stay informed:

1. Subscribe to reputable dementia care newsletters
2. Follow leading dementia organizations on social media
3. Join online forums or support groups for caregivers
4. Read books and articles by dementia care experts
5. Consult regularly with healthcare professionals involved in your loved one's care

Resource Type	Examples	Benefits
Newsletters	Alzheimer's Association, Dementia Society of America	Regular updates on research and care techniques
Online Forums	Alzheimer's Association ALZConnected, Dementia Talking Point	Peer support and shared experiences
Books	"The 36-Hour Day" by Nancy L. Mace and Peter V. Rabins	In-depth knowledge and practical advice

Attending workshops and seminars

Workshops and seminars offer valuable opportunities to learn from experts, connect with other caregivers, and gain hands-on experience with new care techniques. Consider the following when seeking out educational opportunities:

- Look for local events hosted by hospitals, community centers, or dementia care organizations
- Explore online webinars and virtual conferences for convenient learning options

- Attend caregiver support group meetings that often feature educational components
- Investigate training programs offered by local hospice or home health agencies
- Consider certification programs in dementia care if you're looking for more comprehensive education

Remember, investing time in these educational opportunities benefits your loved one and is an act of self-care that can boost your confidence and reduce stress in your caregiving role.

Developing patience and communication skills

Caring for someone with dementia requires extraordinary patience and effective communication skills. These abilities don't always come naturally but can be developed and improved over time. Here are some strategies to enhance these crucial skills:

1. Practice mindfulness and deep breathing to stay calm in challenging situations
2. Learn about the stages of dementia to better understand and anticipate your loved one's needs
3. Use non-verbal communication techniques, such as maintaining eye contact and using a gentle touch
4. Speak clearly and slowly, using simple language and short sentences
5. Develop strategies for redirecting and de-escalating challenging behaviors

Skill	Importance	Development Strategies
Patience	Reduces stress and improves quality of care	Practice mindfulness, take regular breaks, seek support when needed
Communication	It enhances understanding and reduces frustration	Learn about non-verbal cues, practice active listening, and adjust your speaking style
Empathy	Builds trust and strengthens your relationship	Try to see situations from your loved one's perspective, and join a support group to share experiences.

Developing these skills takes time and practice. Be patient with yourself as you learn and grow in your caregiving role. Remember that every caregiver faces challenges, and it's okay to make mistakes. What's important is your commitment to learning and improving.

By staying informed about dementia care techniques, attending educational events, and continually developing your patience and communication skills, you can improve your care and take important steps to prevent burnout and maintain your well-being.

Your dedication to learning and growing as a caregiver is admirable. It reflects the depth of your commitment to your loved one and personal growth. As you continue on this journey, remember that every new skill you acquire and every bit of knowledge you gain is a valuable tool in your caregiving toolkit, helping you navigate the challenges of dementia care with greater confidence and compassion.

Planning: Legal and Financial Considerations

Taking care of a loved one with dementia is a journey that requires both compassion and preparation. As you embark on this path, addressing legal and financial matters early on is not just important; it's a responsibility. This proactive approach can save you from stress and complications, allowing you to focus on what truly matters - providing love and care for your loved one with dementia.

Understanding the Importance of Early Planning

Early planning is not just a precaution; it's a necessity. When your loved one is in the early stages of dementia, they may still have the mental capacity to make crucial decisions and express their wishes. By addressing legal and financial matters early, you:

- Ensure your loved one's voice is heard in future care decisions
- Protect their assets and finances
- Reduce potential family conflicts
- Gain peace of mind for both you and your loved one

Remember, dementia is progressive. There may come a time when your family member can no longer make sound decisions or sign legal documents. **Acting early puts you in the best position to honor their wishes and manage their care effectively.**

Financial and Legal Considerations

Navigating caregiving's financial and legal aspects can be overwhelming for a caregiver. However, understanding these elements is crucial for ensuring the best care for your loved one and protecting your financial well-being. Let's explore the key areas you need to consider.

Planning for Long-Term Care Expenses

Long-term care can be costly, and planning to manage these expenses effectively is essential. Here are some steps to help you prepare:

1. **Assess Current and Future Needs**
    - Evaluate your loved one's current health status and potential future needs
    - Consider the possibility of in-home care, assisted living, or nursing home care

2. **Estimate Costs**
    - Research the costs of different care options in your area
    - Factor in potential increases in healthcare costs over time

3. **Review Available Resources**
    - Assess your loved one's savings, assets, and income sources
    - Consider potential family contributions

4. **Explore Insurance Options**
    - Look into long-term care insurance policies
    - Understand what Medicare and Medicaid may cover

5. **Consult Financial Professionals**
    - Speak with a financial advisor experienced in elder care planning
    - Consider meeting with an elder law attorney

Long-Term Care Funding Options:

- Personal savings and assets
- Long-term care insurance
- Life insurance policies with long-term care riders
- Reverse mortgages (for homeowners)

- Veterans benefits (for eligible veterans and their spouses)
- Medicaid (for those who qualify based on financial need)

Care Type	Average Monthly Cost (2024)	Potential Funding Sources
In-Home Care (44 hours/week)	$4,000 - $8,000	Personal funds, LTC insurance, Medicaid waivers
Assisted Living Facility	$4,500 - $7,000	Personal funds, LTC insurance, some Medicaid programs
Nursing Home (Semi-Private Room)	$7,000 - $14,000	Medicare (short-term), Medicaid, personal funds, LTC insurance
Nursing Home (Private Room)	$8,000 - $15,000	Medicare (short-term), Medicaid, personal funds, LTC insurance
Adult Day Health Care	$1,800 - $2,600	Medicaid waivers, personal funds, some LTC insurance policies

Understanding Legal Rights and Options

Navigating the legal aspects of caregiving is crucial for protecting your loved one's interests and ensuring their wishes are respected. Here are critical legal considerations:

1. **Advance Directives**
    - Encourage your loved one to create or update their advance directives
    - Ensure you have copies of living wills and healthcare power of attorney documents

2. **Power of Attorney**
    - Understand the difference between medical and financial power of attorney
    - Consider setting up a durable power of attorney for finances and healthcare
3. **Guardianship/Conservatorship**
    - Know when these might be necessary and how to pursue them if needed
    - Understand the responsibilities and limitations of these roles
4. **Estate Planning**
    - Encourage your loved one to create or update their will
    - Discuss options like trusts for managing assets
5. **HIPAA Authorization**
    - Ensure you have the necessary authorization to access your loved one's medical information

Essential Legal Documents for Caregivers:

- Durable Power of Attorney for Healthcare
- Durable Power of Attorney for Finances
- Living Will
- HIPAA Authorization Form
- Will and Trust Documents
- Do Not Resuscitate (DNR) Order (if applicable)

Legal Document	Purpose	When to Obtain
Healthcare Power of Attorney	Designates someone to make medical decisions if the person is incapacitated	As early as possible while the person can make sound decisions
Financial Power of Attorney	Allows the designated person to manage finances	Before the cognitive decline, update as needed
Living Will	Specifies end-of-life care preferences	When creating advance directives, review them periodically
HIPAA Authorization	Allows access to medical information	When beginning the caregiving role, update annually

Medical Power of Attorney: What It Is and Why It Matters

A Medical Power of Attorney (MPOA) is a legal document that allows your loved one to appoint someone they trust to make healthcare decisions on their behalf if they cannot do so themselves. This person is often called a healthcare proxy or agent.

Why is an MPOA crucial?

1. It ensures medical decisions align with your loved one's wishes
2. It prevents potential disagreements among family members about care
3. It allows for quick decision-making in emergencies
4. It gives healthcare providers a clear point of contact for meaningful discussions

To set up an MPOA:

1. Discuss the role with your loved one and decide who should be the healthcare proxy
2. Consult with an elder law attorney to draft the document
3. Ensure the document is properly signed and witnessed
4. Provide copies to healthcare providers and family members

Financial Power of Attorney: Protecting Assets and Finances

A Financial Power of Attorney (FPOA) is similar to an MPOA but focuses on financial matters. This document allows your loved one to designate someone to manage their finances if they cannot do so themselves.

Critical aspects of an FPOA:

- It can be immediate or "springing" (only taking effect under specific circumstances)
- It can be broad or limited in scope
- It ends upon the death of your loved one

Benefits of having an FPOA:

- Ensures bills are paid, and finances are managed properly
- Protects against financial exploitation
- Allows for long-term financial planning
- Provides a clear authority for financial institutions to work with

Living Wills and Advance Directives

A living will, often part of an advance directive, is a document that outlines your loved one's wishes for end-of-life care. It typically covers preferences for:

- Use of life-sustaining treatments
- Pain management and comfort care
- Organ donation

Why are these documents important?

- They provide clear guidance in difficult situations
- They reduce the emotional burden on family members making tough decisions
- They ensure your loved one's wishes are respected, even if they can't communicate

When and How to Have These Conversations

Timing is crucial when discussing these sensitive topics. Here are some tips:

1. Start early, ideally when your loved one is first diagnosed
2. Choose a calm, private setting
3. Include other family members if appropriate
4. Be patient and prepared for multiple conversations

Conversation starters:

- "I know this is hard to discuss, but I want to ensure we honor your wishes."
- "Have you thought about what kind of medical care you'd want if you couldn't make decisions?"
- "I've been reading about the importance of having certain legal documents. Can we talk about that?"

Finding Legal Assistance for Document Preparation

While finding templates for these documents online is possible, **working with an elder law attorney is highly recommended.** They can:

- Ensure documents are correctly prepared and legally binding
- Provide advice on complex family or financial situations
- Help navigate state-specific laws and requirements

To find a qualified attorney:

- Ask for recommendations from your local Alzheimer's Association chapter
- Contact your state or local bar association
- Look for attorneys certified in elder law by the National Elder Law Foundation

Proper legal preparation can save significant future stress, time, and money.

Document	Purpose	Key Points
Medical Power of Attorney	Designates someone to make healthcare decisions	• Choose a trusted individual • Discuss preferences in advance • Provide copies to healthcare providers
Financial Power of Attorney	Allows someone to manage finances	• Can be immediate or "springing" • Protects against financial exploitation • Ends upon death
Living Will/Advance Directive	Outlines end-of-life care preferences	• Covers life-sustaining treatments • Addresses pain management • Includes organ donation wishes

By addressing these legal and financial considerations early, you're taking a crucial step in ensuring the best possible care for your loved one with dementia. Remember, you're not alone in this journey. Seek support from professionals, support groups, and your community as you navigate this challenging but essential process.

Exploring Financial Assistance Programs

Various programs and resources are available to help ease the financial burden of caregiving. Here's an overview of potential assistance options:

1. **Government Programs**
    - Medicare: Understand coverage for hospital stays, doctor visits, and some home healthcare
    - Medicaid: Explore eligibility for long-term care coverage
    - Social Security Disability Insurance (SSDI): For those under 65 with qualifying disabilities
    - Supplemental Security Income (SSI): For low-income individuals with disabilities

2. **Veterans Benefits**
    - Aid and Attendance benefits for veterans and surviving spouses
    - Veteran-Directed Care Program
    - VA Caregiver Support Program

3. **State and Local Programs**
    - Area Agencies on Aging: Local resources and support programs
    - State-specific caregiver support programs
    - Respite care grants or vouchers

4. **Non-Profit Organizations**
    - Disease-specific organizations offering financial assistance
    - Local charities and community organizations

5. **Employer Benefits**
   - Check if your employer offers caregiver support or flexible work arrangements
   - Employee Assistance Programs (EAPs) may provide counseling or referrals

6. **Tax Deductions and Credits**
   - Explore potential tax benefits for caregivers
   - Consult a tax professional to understand your eligibility

Steps to Access Financial Assistance:

1. Research programs you might be eligible for
2. Gather necessary documentation (medical records, financial information)
3. Contact program administrators or local offices for application procedures
4. Consider seeking help from a social worker or case manager to navigate options
5. Be persistent and don't hesitate to appeal if initially denied

Assistance Type	Potential Programs	Eligibility Factors
Government Assistance	Medicare, Medicaid, SSDI, SSI	Age, disability status, income, assets
Veterans Benefits	Aid and Attendance, VA Caregiver Support	Military service, disability rating, income
State Programs	Caregiver support, respite care grants	Varies by state, often based on need
Non-Profit Assistance	Disease-specific org grants, local charities	Diagnosis, financial need, location

Remember, navigating caregiving's financial and legal aspects can be complex, but you don't have to do it alone. Don't hesitate to seek professional advice from financial advisors, elder law attorneys, or social workers specializing in senior care. Many communities offer free or low-cost legal clinics and financial counseling services for caregivers.

Addressing these matters early and revisiting them regularly as circumstances change is essential. By understanding and planning for caregiving's financial and legal aspects, you can ensure better care for your loved one and protect your financial well-being.

Understanding and managing these considerations can provide peace of mind, allowing you to focus more energy on the day-to-day aspects of caregiving and your relationship with your loved one. Remember, being proactive in these areas is an integral part of your role as a caregiver and a vital aspect of self-care.

Validation Therapy

Naomi Feil's Validation Therapy

Validation Therapy is a compassionate approach developed by Naomi Feil to help people with dementia feel understood and valued. It involves acknowledging and validating their feelings and experiences rather than trying to correct or dismiss them.

History and Development

Naomi Feil, a social worker, developed validation therapy between 1963 and 1980. She grew up in a family home for seniors and noticed that traditional therapies often upset or isolated elderly patients with dementia. She sought a better way to communicate with them, leading to the creation of Validation Therapy.

Key milestones:

- **1963-1980:** Development of Validation Therapy by Naomi Feil
- **1982:** Publication of Feil's first book on Validation Therapy
- **1980s:** Gained attention in the U.S. through presentations and research

Core Principles

Validation Therapy is based on several core principles guiding caregivers' interactions with dementia patients.

Core principles include:

1. **Acceptance:** Accept the person where they are and where they are not.
2. **Empathy:** Step into their world and feel what they feel.
3. **Respect:** Validate their emotions and experiences without judgment.
4. **Communication:** Use verbal and non-verbal techniques to connect.

Principle	Description
Acceptance	Accept the person as they are
Empathy	Feel what they feel.
Respect	Validate emotions and experiences.
Communication	Use verbal and non-verbal techniques.

Benefits for Dementia Patients

Validation Therapy offers numerous benefits for dementia patients, helping them feel more connected and less isolated.

Benefits include:

- **Restoration of self-worth:** Patients feel valued and understood.
- **Reduced withdrawal:** Encourages interaction with others.
- **Decreased stress and anxiety:** Provides emotional comfort.
- **Improved communication:** Enhances the ability to express feelings.
- **Stimulation of potential:** Helps patients engage in meaningful activities.

Benefit	Description
Restoration of self-worth	Patients feel valued and understood.
Reduced withdrawal	Encourages interaction with others
Decreased stress and anxiety	Provides emotional comfort
Improved communication	Enhances ability to express feelings
Stimulation of potential	Helps patients engage in meaningful activities

Techniques and Examples

Validation Therapy uses specific techniques to connect with dementia patients and validate their feelings.

Techniques include:

- **Mirroring:** Reflecting the patient's body language and emotions.
- **Rephrasing:** Restating what the patient says to show understanding.
- **Reminiscence:** Encouraging patients to talk about past experiences.
- **Touch:** Using gentle touch to convey empathy and support.
- **Eye contact:** Maintaining eye contact to build trust.

Examples of techniques:

1. **Mirroring:**
    - If a patient is wringing their hands, the caregiver might gently mimic this action to show empathy.

2. **Rephrasing:**
    - Patient: "I need to find my mother."
    - Caregiver: "You miss your mother and want to see her."

3. **Reminiscence:**
    - Asking the patient about their favorite childhood memory.

4. **Touch:**
    - Holding the patient's hand during a conversation.

5. **Eye contact:**
    - Looking into the patient's eyes while speaking to them.

Technique	Example
Mirroring	Mimicking hand-wringing to show empathy
Rephrasing	"You miss your mother and want to see her."
Reminiscence	Asking about favorite childhood memory
Touch	Holding the patient's hand
Eye contact	Maintaining eye contact during conversation

Using these techniques, caregivers can create a supportive and understanding environment for dementia patients, helping them feel more secure and less anxious. Validation Therapy is a powerful tool that respects the dignity and emotions of those with dementia, fostering meaningful connections and improving their overall well-being.

Other Validation Techniques

In addition to Naomi Feil's Validation Therapy, several other nonpharmacological methods can be effective in managing dementia symptoms. These methods focus on empathetic communication and creating a supportive environment for dementia patients.

Empathetic Listening

Empathetic listening involves genuinely hearing and understanding what the person with dementia is saying verbally and non-verbally.

Steps for empathetic listening:

1. **Be present:** Give your full attention to the person.
2. **Acknowledge feelings:** Reflect on what you hear to show understanding.
3. **Avoid judgment:** Accept their feelings without trying to correct them.
4. **Use non-verbal cues:** Nod, maintain eye contact, and use appropriate facial expressions.

Example:

- Patient: "I feel so lost."
- Caregiver: "It sounds like you're feeling confused and scared. I'm here with you."

Reassurance and Comfort

Providing reassurance and comfort can help alleviate fear and anxiety in dementia patients.

Ways to provide reassurance:

- **Verbal reassurance:** Use calming and soothing words.
- **Physical comfort:** Offer a gentle touch or a hug.
- **Familiar objects:** Provide comfort items, like a favorite blanket or photo.

Example:

- Patient: "I can't find my way home."
- Caregiver: "You're safe here with me. Let's sit together and talk."

Reminiscence Therapy

Reminiscence therapy involves encouraging dementia patients to talk about their past experiences. This can help them feel more connected and valued.

Benefits of reminiscence therapy:

- **Improves mood:** Talking about happy memories can boost spirits.
- **Enhances communication:** Encourages verbal expression.
- **Strengthens identity:** Helps patients remember who they are.

Techniques for reminiscence therapy:

- **Use photos:** Show old family photos and ask about the people and events in them.
- **Music:** Play songs from their youth and discuss memories associated with the music.
- **Objects:** Use familiar objects to trigger memories and conversations.

Example:

- Caregiver: "Do you remember this photo from your wedding day? Tell me about that day."

Reality Orientation

Reality orientation involves gently reminding dementia patients of the current time, place, and situation to help reduce confusion.

Techniques for reality orientation:

- **Use calendars and clocks:** Place them in visible locations.
- **Daily routines:** Maintain consistent daily schedules.
- **Verbal reminders:** Gently remind them of the date, time, and location.

Example:

- Caregiver: "Good morning, it's Tuesday, June 22nd. We're at home, and it's time for breakfast."

Distraction and Redirection

Distraction and redirection involve shifting the patient's focus from distressing thoughts or behaviors to something more positive.

Techniques for distraction and redirection:

- **Engage in activities:** Suggest a favorite hobby or task.
- **Change the environment:** Move to a different room or walk.
- **Use humor:** Light-hearted jokes or funny stories can help.

Example:

- Patient: "I need to go to work."
- Caregiver: "Let's take a walk in the garden first. Look at these beautiful flowers!"

Cognitive Stimulation Therapy

Cognitive Stimulation Therapy (CST) involves engaging dementia patients in activities that stimulate thinking and memory.

Benefits of CST:

- **Improves cognitive function:** Helps maintain mental abilities.
- **Enhances social interaction:** Encourages group activities and communication.
- **Boosts mood:** Engaging in activities can reduce depression and anxiety.

Examples of CST activities:

- **Puzzles and games:** Crosswords, Sudoku, and memory games.
- **Arts and crafts:** Painting, drawing, and crafting.
- **Group discussions:** Talking about current events or shared interests.

Example:

- Caregiver: "Let's work on this puzzle together. Can you find the corner pieces?"

Environmental Modifications

Modifying the environment can help reduce confusion and agitation in dementia patients.

Tips for environmental modifications:

- **Simplify the space:** Remove clutter and unnecessary items.
- **Use clear signage:** Label rooms and essential items.
- **Ensure safety:** Install grab bars, remove tripping hazards, and use nightlights.

Example:

- Caregiver: "I've labeled the bathroom door and put a nightlight in the hallway to help you find your way at night."

Technique	Description	Example
Empathetic Listening	Genuinely hearing and understanding the patient	"It sounds like you're feeling confused and scared. I'm here with you."
Reassurance and Comfort	Providing verbal and physical comfort	"You're safe here with me. Let's sit together and talk."
Reminiscence Therapy	Encouraging talk about past experiences	"Do you remember this photo from your wedding day? Tell me about that day."
Reality Orientation	Gently reminding of the current time, place, and situation	"Good morning, it's Tuesday, June 22nd. We're at home, and it's time for breakfast."
Distraction and Redirection	Shifting the focus to something positive	"Let's take a walk in the garden first. Look at these beautiful flowers!"
Cognitive Stimulation Therapy	Engaging in activities that stimulate thinking	"Let's work on this puzzle together. Can you find the corner pieces?"
Environmental Modifications	Modifying the environment to reduce confusion	"I've labeled the bathroom door and put a nightlight in the hallway to help you find your way at night."

By using these nonpharmacological methods, caregivers can create a supportive and understanding environment for dementia patients, helping them feel more secure and less anxious. These techniques respect the dignity and emotions of those with dementia, fostering meaningful connections and improving their overall well-being.

Practical Strategies for Caregivers

Caring for someone with dementia can be challenging, but with the right strategies, you can significantly improve their quality of life. Let's explore some practical approaches to help you provide the best care possible.

Identifying and Addressing Unmet Needs

People with dementia may struggle to communicate their needs, leading to frustration and behavioral issues. You can often prevent or reduce challenging behaviors by identifying and addressing these unmet needs.

Common unmet needs to look out for:

- Physical discomfort (pain, hunger, thirst)
- Emotional distress (loneliness, boredom, anxiety)
- Environmental factors (too hot, too cold, too noisy)
- Need for routine or structure

Steps to identify and address unmet needs:

1. **Observe closely:** Watch for changes in behavior or mood.
2. **Keep a log:** Note patterns in behavior and potential triggers.
3. **Check for physical discomfort:** Ensure basic needs (food, water, toileting) are met.
4. **Offer comfort:** Provide reassurance and emotional support.
5. **Adjust the environment:** Make changes to reduce stress or discomfort.

Need	Possible Signs	Potential Solutions
Hunger/Thirst	Agitation, wandering	Offer snacks or drinks regularly
Pain	Grimacing, guarding a body part	Consult with a doctor for pain management
Boredom	Restlessness, repetitive behaviors	Engage in meaningful activities
Overstimulation	Agitation, trying to leave	Create a calm, quiet space

Creating a Safe and Stable Environment

A safe and stable environment can significantly reduce anxiety and confusion for someone with dementia.

Tips for creating a safe environment:

- **Remove hazards:** Clear clutter, secure loose rugs, and remove dangerous items.
- **Enhance visibility:** Use contrasting colors for essential objects and improve lighting.

- **Simplify the space:** Reduce unnecessary furniture and decorations.
- **Use labels:** Clearly label essential rooms and items.
- **Maintain consistency:** Keep furniture arrangements stable and routines predictable.

Creating a dementia-friendly home:

1. **Kitchen:** Lock up hazardous items and use appliances with automatic shut-off features.
2. **Bathroom:** Install grab bars, use non-slip mats, and consider a raised toilet seat.
3. **Bedroom:** Ensure a clear path to the bathroom, and use nightlights.
4. **Living areas:** Remove or secure items that could cause trips or falls.

Communication Tips for De-escalating Fear

Effective communication is critical to managing fear and anxiety in someone with dementia.

General communication tips:

- Speak clearly and slowly
- Use simple language and short sentences
- Maintain eye contact and a calm demeanor
- Use a gentle touch when appropriate

Strategies for de-escalating fear:

1. **Validate feelings:** Acknowledge their emotions without judgment.
    - Example: "I can see you're feeling scared. It's okay, I'm here with you."
2. **Use distraction:** Redirect attention to a pleasant topic or activity.
    - Example: "Let's look at your family photo album together."
3. **Provide reassurance:** Offer comfort and support.
    - Example: "You're safe here. I'll stay with you until you feel better."
4. **Create a calm environment:** Reduce noise and distractions.
    - Example: Turn off the TV, close curtains, or move to a quieter room.
5. **Use visual cues:** Show, don't just tell.
    - Example: If it's time for a meal, show them the table set with food.

De-escalation techniques:

Technique	Description	Example
Validation	Acknowledge feelings	"I understand you're feeling upset."
Distraction	Redirect attention	"Would you like to help me fold these towels?"
Reassurance	Provide comfort	"You're safe here with me."
Environment	Create calm	Reduce noise, adjust lighting
Visual cues	Show, don't tell	Point to or show objects instead of just describing them

Remember, every person with dementia is unique, and what works for one may not work for another. Be patient, flexible, and willing to try different approaches. Your compassion and understanding can make a world of difference in the life of someone with dementia.

Case Studies and Real-Life Examples

Understanding how different approaches work in real-life situations can be incredibly helpful for caregivers. Here, we will explore success stories with Validation Therapy and how combining pharmacological and nonpharmacological approaches can be effective.

Success Stories with Validation Therapy

Validation Therapy has been used successfully in many cases to improve the quality of life for dementia patients. Here are a few examples:

Case Study 1: Mrs. Johnson

Background:

- Mrs. Johnson, an 85-year-old woman with Alzheimer's disease, frequently called out for her deceased mother, causing distress to herself and her caregivers.

Approach:

- Caregivers used Validation Therapy by acknowledging her feelings and gently engaging her in conversations about her mother.

Outcome:

- Mrs. Johnson became calmer and more content. She started sharing happy memories about her mother, which reduced her anxiety and agitation.

Case Study 2: Mr. Smith

Background:

- Mr. Smith, a 78-year-old man with Lewy body dementia, often saw imaginary animals in his room, leading to fear and confusion.

Approach:

- Caregivers used Validation Therapy by acknowledging his fear and gently redirecting his attention to a favorite activity, like listening to music.

Outcome:

- Mr. Smith's episodes of fear decreased, and he became more engaged in activities he enjoyed, improving his overall mood.

Case Study	Background	Approach	Outcome
Mrs. Johnson	Called out for deceased mother	Acknowledged feelings, engaged in conversations about mother	Reduced anxiety and agitation
Mr. Smith	Saw imaginary animals	Acknowledged fear, redirected to a favorite activity	Decreased fear, improved mood

By using these nonpharmacological methods, caregivers can create a supportive and understanding environment for dementia patients, helping them feel more secure and less anxious. These techniques respect the dignity and emotions of those with dementia, fostering meaningful connections and improving their overall well-being.

Nutrition and Dementia

Understanding Eating Challenges in Dementia

As a caregiver or family member of someone with dementia, it's crucial to understand how the progression of the disease can affect your loved one's eating habits and nutritional status. This knowledge will help you provide better care and support throughout your journey.

How Dementia Progression Affects Appetite and Eating Habits

Dementia can impact eating habits in various ways as the disease progresses:

1. **Early Stage:**
    - Subtle changes in taste and smell
    - Difficulty with complex meal planning and preparation
    - Occasional forgetfulness about meals
2. **Middle Stage:**
    - Increased difficulty with utensils
    - Distractibility during meals
    - Changes in food preferences
    - Difficulty recognizing food items
3. **Late Stage:**
    - Significant swallowing difficulties (dysphagia)
    - Inability to feed oneself
    - Refusal to eat or drink
    - Loss of appetite

Fundamental Changes Throughout Progression:

- **Sensory Changes:** Altered taste and smell perception can lead to decreased enjoyment of food.
- **Cognitive Decline:** Forgetting to eat, inability to express hunger, or difficulty recognizing food.
- **Motor Skills:** Challenges using utensils or bringing food to the mouth.
- **Behavioral Issues:** Agitation, wandering, or refusal to eat.

Recognizing Signs of Nutritional Issues in Your Loved One

It's essential to be vigilant and watch for signs that may indicate nutritional problems in your loved one with dementia. Here are some key indicators to look out for:

Physical Signs:

- Unexplained weight loss
- Ill-fitting clothes
- Weakness or fatigue
- Dry skin or hair
- Slow wound healing

Behavioral Signs:

- Refusing to eat
- Spitting out food
- Holding food in the mouth
- Increased agitation around mealtimes
- Difficulty swallowing or choking on food

Cognitive Signs:

- Forgetting how to use utensils
- Inability to recognize food items
- Confusion about mealtime routines

Common Nutritional Issues and Their Potential Causes

Nutritional Issue	Potential Causes
Weight Loss	Decreased appetite, forgetting to eat, increased energy expenditure
Dehydration	Forgetting to drink, inability to recognize thirst, swallowing difficulties
Vitamin Deficiencies	Limited food variety, poor absorption, medication interactions
Malnutrition	A combination of factors, including cognitive decline, physical limitations, and sensory changes

Essential Tips for Caregivers:

1. Monitor your loved one's weight regularly.
2. Keep a food diary to track eating habits and preferences.
3. Observe mealtime behaviors and note any changes.
4. Consult with a healthcare professional if you notice persistent issues.
5. Be patient and understanding, as eating challenges can frustrate you and your loved ones.

Remember, early recognition of nutritional issues can lead to better management and improved quality of life for your loved one with dementia. By staying informed and attentive, you can provide the best possible care and support throughout their dementia journey.

The Role of Nutrition in Brain Health

As a caregiver or family member of someone with dementia, understanding the crucial role of nutrition in brain health can significantly impact your loved one's quality of life. Proper nutrition supports overall health, can help maintain cognitive function, and can potentially slow the progression of dementia symptoms.

Essential Vitamins and Minerals for Cognitive Function

The brain requires a variety of nutrients to function optimally. Here are some essential vitamins and minerals that play vital roles in cognitive health:

1. **B-Complex Vitamins** are crucial for brain function and energy metabolism.
2. **Vitamin C**: A powerful antioxidant that protects brain cells from damage.
3. **Vitamin D3**: Important for neurotransmitter function and neuroprotection.
4. **Vitamin K2**: Supports brain cell membrane health and cognitive function.
5. **Omega-3 Fatty Acids**: Essential for brain structure and function.

Let's explore these in more detail and discuss how to incorporate them into daily meals.

Vitamin B Complex

B vitamins are essential for brain health, particularly B6, B9 (folate), and B12. They help:

- Produce neurotransmitters
- Maintain myelin sheaths around nerves
- Reduce homocysteine levels, which can damage brain cells

Incorporating B vitamins into meals:

- Lean meats, fish, and poultry
- Eggs and dairy products
- Leafy green vegetables
- Legumes and whole grains

Tip: Consider a B-complex supplement if your loved one has difficulty absorbing these vitamins from food, which is common in older adults.

Vitamins C, D3, and K2

These vitamins work together to support brain health in various ways:

Vitamin C:

- Powerful antioxidant protecting brain cells from oxidative stress
- Supports the production of neurotransmitters

Vitamin D3:

- Helps regulate neurotransmitter function
- Supports immune function in the brain
- May help clear beta-amyloid plaques associated with Alzheimer's disease

Vitamin K2:

- Supports brain cell membrane health
- May help prevent cognitive decline

Incorporating these vitamins into meals:

1. Vitamin C:
    - Citrus fruits
    - Berries
    - Bell peppers
    - Broccoli and Brussels sprouts
2. Vitamin D3:
    - Fatty fish (salmon, mackerel)
    - Egg yolks
    - Fortified foods
    - Sun exposure (with caution)
3. Vitamin K2:
    - Fermented foods (natto, sauerkraut)
    - Grass-fed dairy products
    - Egg yolks
    - Organ meats

Note: Vitamin D3 and K2 supplements may be necessary, especially for those with limited sun exposure or dietary restrictions. Always consult with a healthcare provider before starting any supplement regimen.

Omega-3 Fatty Acids

Omega-3s, particularly DHA and EPA, are crucial for brain health:

- Form a significant portion of brain cell membranes
- Support neurotransmitter function
- Have anti-inflammatory properties
- May help reduce the risk of cognitive decline and dementia

Incorporating Omega-3s into meals:

- Fatty fish (salmon, sardines, mackerel) at least twice a week
- Walnuts and flaxseeds
- Chia seeds
- Algae-based supplements for vegetarians/vegans

Brain-Boosting Nutrients and Their Food Sources

Nutrient	Food Sources	Benefits of Brain Health
B-Complex Vitamins	Lean meats, eggs, leafy greens	Neurotransmitter production, nerve health
Vitamin C	Citrus fruits, berries, bell peppers	Antioxidant protection, neurotransmitter support
Vitamin D3	Fatty fish, egg yolks, sunlight	Neurotransmitter regulation, neuroprotection
Vitamin K2	Fermented foods, grass-fed dairy	Brain cell membrane health
Omega-3 Fatty Acids	Fatty fish, walnuts, flaxseeds	Brain structure and function, anti-inflammatory

Tips for Incorporating Brain-Boosting Nutrients into Daily Meals

1. **Plan balanced meals:** Include a variety of colorful fruits and vegetables, lean proteins, and healthy fats in each meal.
2. **Make smoothies:** Blend berries, leafy greens, and chia seeds for a nutrient-packed drink.
3. **Use herbs and spices:** Many herbs, like turmeric and rosemary, have neuroprotective properties.
4. **Choose whole grains:** For B vitamins and fiber, use brown rice, quinoa, and whole wheat bread.
5. **Snack smartly:** Offer nuts, seeds, and fresh fruits as nutritious snacks.

While nutrition is crucial, it's just one aspect of dementia care. For the best results, combine a brain-healthy diet with regular physical activity, social engagement, and cognitive stimulation. Always consult healthcare professionals before significantly changing your loved one's diet or starting any new supplement regimen.

By focusing on these brain-boosting nutrients and incorporating them into daily meals, you're taking an essential step in supporting your loved one's cognitive health and overall well-being. Your dedication to their care is admirable; these nutritional strategies can be a powerful tool in your caregiving journey.

Supplements and Alternative Nutrition Sources

As a caregiver or family member of someone with dementia, you're likely always on the lookout for ways to support your loved one's cognitive health and overall well-being. While a balanced diet is crucial, supplements and alternative nutrition may offer additional benefits. Let's explore three promising options: Lion's Mane Mushroom, Magnesium Glycinate, and MCT oil.

Lion's Mane Mushroom: Benefits for Mood and Cognition

Lion's Mane mushroom, scientifically known as Hericium erinaceus, has gained attention for its potential cognitive benefits.

Key Benefits:

1. **Neurotrophic Properties:** May stimulate the growth of brain cells
2. **Cognitive Support:** Potential to improve memory and focus
3. **Mood Enhancement:** This may help reduce symptoms of anxiety and depression
4. **Neuroprotective Effects:** Possible protection against neurodegenerative diseases

How to Incorporate Lion's Mane:

- Supplements (capsules or powders)
- Teas or coffee blends
- Culinary use in dishes (when available fresh)

Caution: While considered safe, consult a healthcare provider before starting any new supplement, especially if your loved one takes medications.

Magnesium Glycinate: Supporting Brain Health and Relaxation

Magnesium is an essential mineral crucial to brain health and overall bodily function. Magnesium Glycinate is a well-absorbed form and may have additional benefits for cognitive function and relaxation.

Key Benefits:

1. **Cognitive Support:** May improve memory and learning
2. **Stress Reduction:** This can help promote relaxation and reduce anxiety
3. **Sleep Improvement:** May enhance sleep quality
4. **Neuroprotection:** Potential to protect brain cells from damage

How to Incorporate Magnesium Glycinate:

- Supplements (capsules or powders)
- Topical magnesium oils or lotions
- Foods high in magnesium (though Glycinate form is mainly available as a supplement)

Magnesium-Rich Foods

Food	Magnesium Content (per 100g)
Pumpkin seeds	592 mg
Almonds	270 mg
Spinach	79 mg
Dark chocolate	228 mg
Avocado	29 mg

Note: While these foods are excellent sources of magnesium, they may not provide the specific benefits of Magnesium Glycinate. Consult with a healthcare provider about supplementation.

MCT Oil: A Potential Brain Fuel Source

Medium-chain triglyceride (MCT) oil has gained popularity for its potential cognitive benefits, particularly in the context of dementia and Alzheimer's disease.

Key Benefits:

1. **Alternative Brain Fuel:** May provide ketones as an energy source for brain cells
2. **Cognitive Function:** Potential to improve memory and cognitive performance
3. **Neuroprotection:** Possible protective effects against neurodegeneration
4. **Mood Support:** May help stabilize mood and reduce anxiety

How to Incorporate MCT Oil:

1. **Add to beverages:**
   - Mix into coffee or tea
   - Blend into smoothies
2. **Use in cooking:**
   - Drizzle over salads
   - Use in low-heat cooking (not suitable for high-heat frying)
3. **Supplement form:**
   - Capsules or liquid supplements

Important Considerations:

- Start with small amounts (1 teaspoon) and gradually increase to avoid digestive discomfort
- Choose high-quality, pure MCT oil
- Consult with a healthcare provider before starting MCT oil, especially if your loved one has diabetes or liver issues

Comparison of Supplement Options

Supplement	Primary Benefits	Form	Potential Side Effects
Lion's Mane Mushroom	Cognitive support, mood enhancement	Capsules, powders, teas	Rare; may include digestive issues
Magnesium Glycinate	Relaxation, sleep improvement, cognitive support	Capsules, powders, topical	Rare; may include digestive issues at high doses
MCT Oil	Alternative brain fuel, cognitive function	Liquid oil, capsules	Digestive discomfort if introduced too quickly

General Tips for Incorporating Supplements:

1. **Always consult a healthcare provider** before starting any new supplement regimen.
2. **Start with low doses** and gradually increase to assess tolerance.
3. **Monitor for any changes** in mood, behavior, or cognitive function.
4. **Be patient** - benefits may take weeks or months to become noticeable.
5. **Keep a journal** to track any improvements or side effects.
6. **Remember that supplements are not a cure** but may offer supportive benefits.

As a caregiver, your dedication to exploring options for supporting your loved one's health is commendable. While these supplements and alternative nutrition sources show promise, it's essential to approach them as part of a comprehensive care plan that includes a balanced diet, regular exercise, social engagement, and ongoing medical care.

Everyone is unique, and what works for one person may not work for another. Your attentiveness to your loved one's needs and responses is invaluable in finding the most effective approach to supporting their cognitive health and overall well-being.

Encouraging Independent Eating and Drinking

As a caregiver or family member of someone with dementia, maintaining your loved one's independence during mealtimes is crucial for their dignity and self-esteem. Encouraging self-feeding can also help preserve motor skills and cognitive function. Let's explore how to create a supportive environment and promote independent eating and drinking for as long as possible.

Creating a Supportive Mealtime Environment

The right environment can significantly impact your loved one's ability and willingness to eat independently. Here are vital factors to consider:

1. **Minimize distractions:**
   - Turn off the TV and reduce background noise
   - Clear the table of unnecessary items
   - Use simple, solid-colored placemats to reduce visual confusion
2. **Ensure proper lighting:**
   - Provide adequate, non-glare lighting
   - Avoid shadows that might cause confusion or misperception
3. **Create a calm atmosphere:**
   - Play soft, soothing music if it helps your loved one relax
   - Speak in a gentle, encouraging tone
   - Avoid rushing or pressuring your loved one to eat quickly
4. **Establish a routine:**
   - Serve meals at consistent times each day
   - Use familiar plates, utensils, and seating arrangements
5. **Promote social interaction:**
   - Eat together when possible
   - Engage in light, pleasant conversation during meals

Elements of a Supportive Mealtime Environment

Element	Purpose	Examples
Minimal Distractions	Improve focus and reduce confusion	Turn off the TV, clear unnecessary items
Proper Lighting	Enhance visibility and reduce misperceptions	Use non-glare lighting, avoid shadows
Calm Atmosphere	Reduce anxiety and promote relaxation	Play soft music, speak gently
Consistent Routine	Provide structure and familiarity	Regular mealtimes, familiar tableware
Social Interaction	Encourage engagement and enjoyment	Eat together, engage in light conversation

Practical Tips for Promoting Self-Feeding

Encouraging independence during meals can help maintain your loved one's skills and confidence. Here are some practical strategies:

1. **Simplify the table setting:**
   - Use contrasting colors for plates and tablecloths to make food more visible
   - Provide only necessary utensils to reduce confusion
2. **Adapt utensils and dishes:**
   - Use plates with high sides or bowls to prevent spills
   - Provide utensils with larger, easier-to-grip handles
   - Consider weighted utensils to reduce hand tremors
3. **Serve finger foods:**
   - Cut food into bite-sized pieces
   - Offer foods that are easy to pick up and eat without utensils
4. **Provide verbal cues and gentle reminders:**
   - Use simple, step-by-step instructions if needed
   - Offer gentle reminders to continue eating if your loved one becomes distracted
5. **Allow extra time for meals:**
   - Be patient and avoid rushing
   - Plan for longer mealtimes to reduce stress
6. **Encourage hydration:**
   - Keep drinks within easy reach
   - Use cups with lids and straws to prevent spills

7. **Respect food preferences:**
   - Offer favorite foods when possible
   - Be mindful of texture preferences and any swallowing difficulties

When and How to Offer Assistance

While promoting independence is essential, there may come a time when your loved one needs more help during meals. Here's how to recognize when assistance is required and how to provide it respectfully:

Signs that aid may be necessary:

- Difficulty manipulating utensils
- Forgetting to eat or drink
- Becoming easily frustrated during meals
- Significant weight loss or dehydration

How to offer assistance:

1. **Start with minimal intervention:**
   - Sit next to your loved one and eat together
   - Demonstrate eating motions to encourage mimicking
2. **Use hand-over-hand guidance:**
   - Gently place your hand over theirs to guide utensils to their mouth
   - Gradually reduce assistance as they regain the motion
3. **Offer verbal prompts and encouragement:**
   - Use clear, simple instructions: "Pick up your fork," "Take a bite."
   - Offer praise and encouragement for their efforts
4. **Alternate between assistance and independence:**
   - Help with more challenging foods but allow independence with more accessible items
   - Encourage self-feeding for as long as possible during the meal
5. **Maintain dignity:**
   - Avoid treating your loved one like a child
   - Respect their preferences and pace
6. **Be flexible:**
   - Adapt your approach based on your loved one's changing needs
   - Some days may require more assistance than others

Remember: The goal is to support your loved one's independence while ensuring they receive adequate nutrition and hydration. This delicate balance may change over time.

Levels of Mealtime Assistance

Level of Assistance	When to Use	Examples
Minimal Intervention	Early stages or good days	Eating together, gentle reminders
Moderate Assistance	Increasing difficulty but some independence	Hand-over-hand guidance, verbal prompts
Full Assistance	Significant difficulty, safety concerns	Feeding your loved one, ensuring proper positioning

As a caregiver, your patience and understanding during mealtimes are invaluable. Remember that each day may differ, and adjusting your approach as needed is okay. Your efforts to maintain your loved one's dignity and independence during meals profoundly express care and respect.

By creating a supportive environment, encouraging self-feeding, and offering assistance when necessary, you're not just providing nutrition – you're preserving your loved one's sense of self and quality of life. Your dedication to this aspect of care is truly admirable.

Understanding and Managing Swallowing Difficulties (Dysphagia)

As a caregiver or family member of someone with dementia, you may encounter challenges related to swallowing difficulties, known medically as dysphagia. Understanding this condition and learning how to manage it is crucial for ensuring your loved one's safety, nutrition, and quality of life.

What is Dysphagia, and How Does it Progress in Dementia?

Dysphagia is a term used to describe difficulty or discomfort in swallowing. In the context of dementia, dysphagia often develops as the disease progresses, affecting the complex neurological processes involved in swallowing.

Progression of Dysphagia in Dementia:

1. **Early Stage:**
   - Occasional coughing or throat clearing during meals
   - Slight difficulty with certain textures
2. **Middle Stage:**
   - More frequent coughing or choking during meals
   - Difficulty managing mixed textures
   - Pocketing food in cheeks
3. **Late Stage:**
   - Significant difficulty swallowing both solids and liquids
   - Frequent coughing, choking, or aspiration
   - Inability to manage own feeding

Critical Signs of Dysphagia:

- Coughing or choking during or after eating
- Wet or gurgling voice after swallowing
- Difficulty initiating a swallow
- Food or liquid leaking from the mouth
- Unexplained weight loss or dehydration
- Recurrent chest infections or pneumonia

Understanding the risks:

Dysphagia can lead to severe complications, including:

- Aspiration pneumonia
- Malnutrition
- Dehydration
- Decreased quality of life

Adapting Food Textures and Liquid Consistencies

As dysphagia progresses, it's essential to adapt the textures of foods and the consistency of liquids to make swallowing safer and more accessible for your loved one.

Food Texture Modifications:

1. **Regular:** Normal textures, no modifications needed
2. **Soft:** Cooked until tender, can be cut with a fork
3. **Minced and Moist:** Finely chopped or ground, moist and soft
4. **Pureed:** Smooth, lump-free consistency

Liquid Consistency Modifications:

1. **Thin:** Regular liquids (water, tea, coffee)
2. **Slightly Thick:** Easily pourable, coats the back of a spoon
3. **Mildly Thick:** Pours slowly, like nectar
4. **Moderately Thick:** Spoonable, like honey
5. **Extremely Thick:** Holds its shape on a spoon, like pudding

Food and Liquid Consistency Progression

Stage	Food Texture	Liquid Consistency	Examples
Early	Soft	Thin to Slightly Thick	Tender meats, cooked vegetables, regular drinks
Middle	Minced and Moist	Mildly to Moderately Thick	Ground meats, mashed vegetables, thickened juices
Late	Pureed	Moderately to Extremely Thick	Smooth purees, puddings, very thick smoothies

Preparing Meals for Different Stages of Dysphagia

Adapting meals to the appropriate texture is crucial for safe and comfortable eating. Here are some tips for preparing meals at different stages of dysphagia: **1. Soft Diet:**

- Cook meats until tender and moist
- Steam or boil vegetables until soft
- Offer soft fruits like ripe bananas or canned fruits

2. Minced and Moist Diet:

- Use a food processor to chop meats and vegetables finely
- Ensure foods are moist by adding gravy or sauce
- Mash foods like potatoes or cooked beans

3. Pureed Diet:

- Blend foods until smooth, adding liquid as needed
- Strain to remove any lumps
- Use thickeners to achieve the right consistency

Tips for All Stages:

- Avoid mixed textures (e.g., soup with chunks)
- Serve foods at a comfortable temperature
- Present foods separately on the plate for visual appeal

Thickening Liquids:

- Use commercial thickeners according to package instructions
- Natural thickeners like mashed banana or yogurt can be used for some beverages

Sample Menu for Pureed Diet:

Meal	Menu Items
Breakfast	Smooth oatmeal, pureed fruit, thickened juice
Lunch	Pureed chicken, mashed potatoes, pureed carrots
Dinner	Pureed fish, pureed spinach, smooth applesauce

Important Safety Considerations:

1. **Consult professionals:** Work with a speech therapist or dietitian to determine the appropriate food textures and liquid consistencies.
2. **Monitor for changes:** Regularly assess your loved one's swallowing abilities, which may change over time.
3. **Maintain good oral hygiene:** This helps prevent bacteria from entering the lungs if aspiration occurs.
4. **Ensure proper positioning:** Have your loved one sit upright during meals and for 30 minutes afterward.

5. **Be patient:** Allow plenty of time for meals to reduce stress and the risk of choking.
6. **Stay alert:** Watch for signs of choking or aspiration during meals.
7. **Encourage independence:** When safe, allow your loved one to feed themselves to maintain dignity and function.

Remember, managing dysphagia is a journey that requires patience, adaptability, and compassion. Your efforts to provide safe, nutritious meals are invaluable to your loved one's health and quality of life. Don't hesitate to seek support from healthcare professionals or support groups as you navigate this aspect of care.

By understanding dysphagia and adapting meals appropriately, you're not just addressing a medical need – you're showing deep care and respect for your loved one's comfort and well-being. Your dedication to this challenging aspect of care is truly admirable.

Preventing Complications: Aspiration Pneumonia

As a caregiver or family member of someone with dementia, understanding and preventing aspiration pneumonia is crucial for your loved one's health and well-being. This condition can be severe, but you can significantly reduce the risks with proper knowledge and care.

Recognizing the Risks of Aspiration

Aspiration occurs when food, liquids, or saliva enter the lungs instead of the stomach. For individuals with dementia, several factors increase the risk of aspiration:

1. **Dysphagia (swallowing difficulties):** Common in later stages of dementia
2. **Reduced cough reflex:** May not clear the airway effectively
3. **Impaired cognitive function:** Difficulty recognizing food or remembering how to chew and swallow
4. **Medications:** Some may cause drowsiness or relax the throat muscles
5. **Poor oral hygiene:** Increases harmful bacteria in the mouth

Signs that may indicate aspiration risk:

- Coughing or choking during meals
- Gurgling or "wet" voice after eating or drinking
- Difficulty managing saliva
- Frequent throat-clearing
- Unexplained fever or respiratory infections

Strategies to Minimize Aspiration During Meals

Implementing these strategies can help reduce the risk of aspiration:

1. **Proper positioning**
    - Ensure your loved one is sitting upright at a 90-degree angle during meals
    - Keep them in an upright position for at least 30 minutes after eating
2. **Food and drink modifications**
    - Thicken liquids as recommended by a speech therapist
    - Cut food into small, manageable pieces
    - Avoid mixed textures (e.g., soup with chunks)
3. **Feeding techniques**
    - Offer small bites and sips
    - Encourage slow eating and drinking
    - Ensure the mouth is empty before offering more food
4. **Environmental considerations**
    - Minimize distractions during meals
    - Ensure adequate lighting
    - Use contrasting colors for plates and tablecloths to improve food visibility
5. **Oral care**
    - Assist with regular brushing and mouth care
    - Clean dentures daily

Texture Modifications for Aspiration Prevention

Food Type	Safe Modifications	Foods to Avoid
Liquids	Thickened to recommended consistency	Thin liquids, if advised
Meats	Ground or pureed	Tough, stringy meats
Vegetables	Soft-cooked, mashed	Raw, fibrous vegetables
Fruits	Soft, peeled, or pureed	Fruits with skins or seeds
Grains	Soft, well-cooked	Dry, crusty bread

When to Seek Medical Help

It's essential to be vigilant and seek medical attention promptly if you notice:

1. **Sudden onset of:**
    - Coughing or choking that doesn't subside
    - Difficulty breathing or shortness of breath
    - Chest pain
    - Fever (especially if over 101°F or 38.3°C)
2. **Gradual changes such as:**
    - Increased fatigue or weakness
    - Decreased appetite
    - Changes in the color or amount of phlegm
    - Worsening confusion or agitation
3. **Any signs of respiratory distress, including:**
    - Blue tinge to lips or fingernails
    - Rapid breathing
    - Use of accessory muscles to breathe

Remember: Trust your instincts. If you're concerned about your loved one's health, seeking medical advice sooner rather than later is always better.

Preventive Measures

Taking proactive steps can significantly reduce the risk of aspiration pneumonia:

1. **Regular dental check-ups and oral care**
2. **Speech therapy evaluations** to assess swallowing function

3. **Occupational therapy** to improve feeding skills
4. **Medication reviews** with the doctor to minimize side effects
5. **Proper hydration** to keep secretions thin

By implementing these strategies and remaining vigilant, you can play a crucial role in preventing aspiration pneumonia and maintaining your loved one's quality of life. Remember, your dedication to their care significantly affects their well-being. Don't hesitate to contact healthcare professionals for support and guidance as you navigate this aspect of care.

Assisting with Feeding: A Compassionate Approach

As a caregiver or family member of someone with dementia, assisting with feeding can be both challenging and rewarding. Your compassionate approach can make mealtimes more comfortable and enjoyable for your loved one. Let's explore techniques for safe feeding, finding the right balance between encouragement and respect, and understanding non-verbal cues.

Techniques for Safe and Comfortable Feeding

Safety and comfort should be your top priorities when assisting your loved one with feeding. Here are some techniques to help you:

1. **Proper Positioning:**
   - Ensure your loved one is sitting upright at a 90-degree angle
   - Use pillows or cushions for support if needed
   - Position yourself at eye level or slightly below
2. **Pacing:**
   - Offer small bites and allow time to swallow between each
   - Count to five after each swallow before offering the next bite
   - Be patient and avoid rushing
3. **Utensil Use:**
   - Use a spoon rather than a fork for easier feeding

- Consider adaptive utensils with larger handles or angled designs
- Alternate between food and drinks to help with swallowing

4. **Food Presentation:**
   - Offer one type of food at a time to avoid confusion
   - Use contrasting colors between the plate and food for better visibility
   - Ensure food is at a comfortable temperature
5. **Communication:**
   - Describe the food you're offering
   - Provide gentle verbal cues like "open" or "swallow."
   - Maintain eye contact and a calm demeanor

Safe Feeding Techniques

Technique	Purpose	Example
Proper Positioning	Reduce choking risk	Upright at 90-degree angle
Pacing	Allow time for swallowing	Count to five between bites
Utensil Selection	Ease of feeding	Use a spoon instead of a fork
Food Presentation	Improve visibility and reduce confusion	One food type at a time
Communication	Provide guidance and comfort	Gentle verbal cues

Encouraging Eating vs. Forcing Food: Finding the Right Balance

Finding the balance between encouraging your loved one to eat and respecting their autonomy can be challenging. Here are some strategies to help:

1. **Create a positive atmosphere:**
   - Use a gentle, encouraging tone
   - Smile and maintain a calm demeanor
   - Play soft background music if it's soothing for your loved one
2. **Offer choices:**
   - When possible, let your loved one choose between two options
   - Respect food preferences and aversions

3. **Use gentle encouragement:**
   - Offer verbal prompts like "This looks delicious" or "Would you like to try this?"
   - Demonstrate eating to encourage mimicking
4. **Respect refusals:**
   - If your loved one turns their head or closes their mouth, respect this as a "no."
   - Take a break and try again later if needed
5. **Focus on quality, not quantity:**
   - Aim for nutrient-dense foods in smaller portions
   - Consider nutritional supplements if recommended by a healthcare provider
6. **Be flexible:**
   - If your loved one is having a difficult day, consider finger foods or a smoothie
   - Adjust meal times to when they seem most receptive

Remember: Forcing food can lead to choking, aspiration, or a negative association with mealtimes. Always prioritize safety and comfort over finishing a meal.

Reading Non-Verbal Cues for Hunger and Fullness

As dementia progresses, your loved one may have difficulty expressing hunger or fullness verbally. Learning to read non-verbal cues is crucial:

Signs of Hunger:

- Increased alertness or agitation
- Putting hands to mouth
- Chewing motions
- Searching or reaching for food
- Increased focus on others eating

Signs of Fullness or Disinterest in Food:

- Turning head away from food
- Pushing food away or spitting it out
- Closing mouth tightly
- Falling asleep during meals
- Playing with food instead of eating

Non-verbal Cues and Possible Meanings

Non-Verbal Cue	Possible Meaning	Suggested Action
Reaching for food	Hunger	Offer food or assist with feeding
Turning head away	Fullness or disinterest	Take a break or end the meal
Chewing motions	Hunger or readiness to eat	Offer food or continue feeding
Pushing food away	Fullness or dislike of food	Try a different food or end the meal
Increased alertness	Possible hunger	Offer food and observe the response

Additional Tips for Reading Cues:

1. **Observe facial expressions:** Look for signs of enjoyment or discomfort
2. **Monitor body language:** Notice tension or relaxation in their posture
3. **Pay attention to sounds:** Contented sounds may indicate enjoyment, while grunts or groans might signal discomfort
4. **Be aware of time:** If it's been several hours since the last meal, they may be hungry even if they are not showing clear signs

Remember, every individual is unique, and learning your loved one's specific cues may take time. Your attentiveness and patience in this process are invaluable.

Assisting with feeding requires patience, empathy, and keen observation. Your compassionate approach ensures proper nutrition and maintains your loved one's dignity and quality of life. Don't hesitate to seek support from healthcare professionals or support groups as you navigate this aspect of care. Your dedication to nurturing, respectful care during mealtimes is admirable and significantly affects your loved one's well-being.

Nutrition in Late-Stage Dementia

As dementia progresses to its late stages, caregivers and family members face unique challenges in meeting their loved one's nutritional needs. This phase requires a delicate balance between providing nourishment and ensuring comfort. Your role in this process is invaluable, and understanding the complexities of nutrition in late-stage dementia can help you make informed, compassionate decisions.

Addressing Changing Nutritional Needs

In late-stage dementia, nutritional requirements often change due to decreased activity levels, metabolic changes, and the progression of the disease. Here's what you need to know:

1. **Caloric Needs:**
   - Generally decrease due to reduced physical activity
   - May increase if there's significant agitation or wandering
2. **Protein Requirements:**
   - Remain essential to prevent muscle wasting
   - May need to be adjusted based on kidney function
3. **Hydration:**
   - Crucial but often overlooked
   - Dehydration can worsen confusion and increase fall risk
4. **Micronutrients:**
   - Vitamin and mineral needs remain important
   - Deficiencies can impact overall health and cognitive function

Nutritional Considerations in Late-Stage Dementia

Nutrient	Importance	Considerations
Calories	Maintain healthy weight	May need to be reduced; monitor weight
Protein	Prevent muscle wasting	Adjust based on individual needs and kidney function
Fluids	Prevent dehydration	Offer frequently; monitor for signs of dehydration
Vitamins & Minerals	Support overall health	Consider supplements if the diet is limited

Strategies for Meeting Nutritional Needs:

- **Nutrient-dense foods:** Focus on foods that provide maximum nutrition in smaller portions
- **Fortified foods:** Use products enriched with vitamins and minerals
- **Texture modifications:** Adapt food textures to make eating more accessible and safer

- **Frequent, small meals:** Offer 5-6 small meals instead of 3 larger ones
- **Oral nutritional supplements:** Use as recommended by healthcare providers

To Feed or Not to Feed: Balancing Comfort and Nutrition

As dementia reaches its final stages, the question of whether to continue feeding efforts can become a challenging ethical and emotional dilemma. Here are some factors to consider:

Reasons to Continue Feeding Efforts:

- Provides comfort and sensory stimulation
- Maintains social interaction and routine
- May prolong life in some cases

Reasons to Reconsider Aggressive Feeding:

- Risk of aspiration and pneumonia
- Discomfort or distress during feeding
- Aligned with advanced directives or previously expressed wishes

Finding the Right Balance:

1. **Consult healthcare providers:**
   - Discuss the benefits and risks of continued feeding
   - Consider palliative care consultation
2. **Respect advance directives:**
   - Honor previously expressed wishes about end-of-life care
3. **Focus on comfort:**
   - Prioritize comfort over nutritional goals
   - Offer favorite foods in safe textures
4. **Consider alternative methods:**
   - Hand feeding with careful attention to swallowing
   - Use of thickened liquids if recommended
5. **Be flexible:**
   - Adapt approach based on day-to-day changes
   - Allow refusal of food or drink

Remember: There's no one-size-fits-all approach. Your decision should be based on your loved one's circumstances, medical advice, and family values.

Recognizing Hunger Cues When Communication is Limited

In late-stage dementia, verbal communication about hunger or fullness may be severely limited or absent. Recognizing non-verbal cues becomes crucial:

Potential Signs of Hunger:

- Opening mouth when food is presented
- Reaching for or pointing to food
- Increased alertness or agitation around mealtimes
- Making chewing motions

Potential Signs of Disinterest or Fullness:

- Turning head away from food
- Keeping the mouth closed when food is offered
- Pushing away or spilling food
- Falling asleep during meals

Interpreting Non-Verbal Cues

Cue	Possible Meaning	Suggested Action
Opening mouth	Readiness to eat	Offer food
Turning head away	Fullness or disinterest	Pause feeding, try again later
Increased alertness	Possible hunger	Offer food and observe the response
Pushing food away	Fullness or dislike of food	Stop feeding and try different foods later

Strategies for Responding to Cues:

1. **Observe closely:**
    - Pay attention to facial expressions and body language
    - Note any patterns in behavior around mealtimes

2. **Offer food regularly:**
   - Present small amounts of food at regular intervals
   - Allow time for a response before offering more
3. **Use sensory cues:**
   - Let your loved one see and smell the food
   - Gently touch their hand or arm to alert them to the presence of food
4. **Be patient:**
   - Allow plenty of time for meals
   - Don't rush or force-feeding
5. **Monitor overall patterns:**
   - Keep a log of eating behaviors and amounts consumed
   - Share observations with healthcare providers

Navigating nutrition in late-stage dementia is a challenging but crucial aspect of care. Your attentiveness to your loved one's changing needs and nonverbal cues is invaluable. Remember that your goal is to provide comfort and quality of life, not just nutrition. It's normal to feel conflicted or uncertain at times—don't hesitate to seek support from healthcare providers, support groups, or counselors.

Your compassionate care during this difficult time is a profound expression of love and respect for your loved one. Trust your instincts, stay informed, and know your efforts significantly affect your loved one's comfort and well-being.

End-of-Life Nutritional Considerations

As your loved one with dementia approaches the end of life, nutritional considerations shift dramatically. This phase can be emotionally challenging, but understanding the natural processes and focusing on comfort can help you provide the most compassionate care possible.

Understanding Natural Changes in Appetite and Thirst

As death approaches, the body undergoes natural changes that affect appetite and thirst:

1. **Decreased appetite:** This is a normal part of dying.
2. **Reduced thirst:** The body's need for fluids diminishes.

3. **Changes in metabolism:** The body requires less energy.
4. **Altered taste and smell:** These senses may become dulled, making food less appealing.

Remember that these changes are not painful or distressing for your loved one. They are part of the body's natural preparation for shutting down.

The Brain's Role in Appetite and Thirst at End of Life

One of the most crucial points to understand is that **your loved one is not starving**. As death approaches, the brain undergoes significant changes:

- **Appetite regulation:** The brain's hunger and thirst centers shut down.
- **Hormonal changes:** Alterations in hormone levels reduce the feeling of hunger.
- **Neurotransmitter shifts:** These affect the perception of the need for food and water.

Key point: The lack of desire to eat or drink is not causing suffering but is a natural part of the dying process.

The Need for Dehydration in the Dying Process

Counterintuitively, a certain level of dehydration is beneficial in the final stages of life:

- **Fluid reduction:** Helps prevent fluid buildup in the lungs and other tissues.
- **Reduced urine output:** Minimizes the need for toileting, increasing comfort.
- **Natural pain relief:** Dehydration can lead to the release of endorphins, providing natural pain relief.
- **Hastens the dying process:** Prevents unnecessary prolonging of the active dying phase.

Remember: This natural dehydration is not painful and can contribute to a more peaceful passing.

The Pros and Cons of Artificial Nutrition

Deciding whether to use artificial nutrition (tube feeding) or IV fluids is a complex and personal decision. Here's a balanced view:

Pros and Cons of Artificial Nutrition

Pros	Cons
It may prolong life.	It can cause discomfort and complications.
Provides hydration	This may lead to fluid overload and breathing difficulties.
Can deliver medications	Risk of infection at insertion sites
Potentially improves strength temporarily.	May prolong the dying process unnecessarily
It gives family members a sense of "doing something."	Can interfere with the natural, comfortable dying process

Important considerations:

- Consult with palliative care specialists for personalized advice.
- Consider your loved one's previously expressed wishes.
- Weigh the potential benefits against the risks and impact on comfort.

Focusing on Comfort and Quality of Life

In the final stages of dementia, the primary goal shifts to ensuring comfort and quality of life:

1. **Mouth care:**
   - Keep lips and mouth moist with swabs or ice chips.
   - Use lip balm to prevent cracking.
2. **Positioning:**
   - Ensure comfortable positioning to ease breathing.
   - Use pillows for support and to prevent pressure sores.
3. **Sensory comfort:**
   - Play soothing music.
   - Use gentle touch or massage.
   - Maintain a calm, peaceful environment.

4. **Symptom management:**
   - Work with healthcare providers to manage any pain or discomfort.
   - Use medications as prescribed for comfort.
5. **Emotional and spiritual support:**
   - Provide a reassuring presence.
   - Honor spiritual or religious practices critical to your loved one.

Remember: Your presence and loving care are the most important things you can offer now.

Practical Tips for End-of-Life Care

1. **Follow your loved one's cues:**
   - Offer small sips of water or favorite drinks if they show interest.
   - Don't force food or drink if refused.
2. **Use ice chips or frozen treats:**
   - These can provide comfort without the risk of choking.
3. **Focus on favorite flavors:**
   - Use flavored swabs or small tastes of favorite foods for comfort.
4. **Maintain oral hygiene:**
   - Regular mouth care is crucial for comfort.
5. **Communicate with the healthcare team:**
   - Report any signs of discomfort or changes in condition.

Navigating end-of-life care for a loved one with dementia is undoubtedly one of the most challenging experiences you may face. Remember that the natural decrease in appetite and thirst is not causing suffering but is part of the body's preparation for death. You provide comfort, love, and support during this transition.

It's normal to feel a range of emotions during this time. Don't hesitate to seek support for yourself from healthcare providers, counselors, or support groups. Your well-being is important, too.

Your presence and compassionate care are invaluable gifts to your loved one. Trust in the natural process, focus on comfort, and know that your loving attention is the most critical nourishment you can receive at this stage of your life's journey.

Practical Tips for Caregivers

As a caregiver for someone with dementia, planning and preparing meals can be challenging yet rewarding. By focusing on nutritious, dementia-friendly meals, adapting familiar recipes, and creating a positive mealtime atmosphere, you can enhance your loved one's dining experience and overall well-being.

Planning and Preparing Nutritious, Dementia-Friendly Meals

When planning meals for someone with dementia, focusing on nutrition while considering their changing needs and abilities is essential. Here are some practical tips to help you:

1. **Focus on nutrient-dense foods:**
   - Lean proteins (chicken, fish, beans)
   - Colorful fruits and vegetables
   - Whole grains
   - Healthy fats (avocado, nuts, olive oil)
2. **Consider texture and ease of eating:**
   - Soft foods that are easy to chew and swallow
   - Bite-sized pieces to promote independence
   - Moist foods to aid swallowing
3. **Incorporate brain-healthy ingredients:**
   - Omega-3-rich foods (salmon, walnuts, flaxseeds)
   - Antioxidant-rich berries
   - Leafy greens
4. **Plan for variety:**
   - Offer a range of colors and flavors to stimulate appetite
   - Rotate meals to prevent boredom
5. **Prepare meals in advance:**
   - Batch cook and freeze portions for convenience
   - Use slow cookers for easy, nutritious meals

Sample Meal Plan for a Day

Meal	Menu Items	Nutritional Benefits
Breakfast	Oatmeal with berries and nuts	Fiber, antioxidants, healthy fats
Lunch	Vegetable soup with soft-cooked chicken	Hydration, protein, vitamins
Dinner	Baked fish with mashed sweet potato and steamed broccoli	Omega-3s, vitamins, easy to eat
Snacks	Greek yogurt with honey, sliced fruit	Protein, probiotics, natural sugars

Adapting Family Recipes for Easier Consumption

Familiar foods can bring comfort and stimulate appetite. Here's how to adapt family favorites:

1. **Modify textures:**
   - Puree or mash foods to make them easier to swallow
   - Use a food processor to chop meats finely
   - Add gravy or sauce to moisten dry foods
2. **Simplify recipes:**
   - Reduce the number of ingredients
   - Focus on key flavors
3. **Enhance flavors:**
   - Use herbs and spices to compensate for changes in taste perception
   - Add natural sweeteners like honey or fruit purees
4. **Make finger foods:**
   - Transform recipes into bite-sized portions
   - Create easy-to-hold shapes
5. **Increase nutrient density:**
   - Add protein powder to smoothies or soups
   - Incorporate healthy fats like avocado or olive oil

Example: Adapting a Family Lasagna Recipe

- Original: Layered pasta with meat sauce and cheese
- Adapted: Pasta shells filled with ground meat and pureed vegetables, topped with melted cheese

Creating a Positive Mealtime Atmosphere

The environment and atmosphere during meals can significantly impact your loved one's eating experience. Here are tips for creating a positive mealtime setting:

1. **Set the stage:**
   - Use contrasting colors for plates and tablecloths
   - Ensure adequate, non-glare lighting
   - Minimize background noise (turn off the TV, reduce loud conversations)
2. **Establish a routine:**
   - Serve meals at consistent times
   - Use familiar place settings
3. **Encourage independence:**
   - Provide adaptive utensils if needed
   - Serve finger foods when appropriate
4. **Dine together:**
   - Make mealtimes a social event
   - Model eating behaviors
5. **Be patient and flexible:**
   - Allow plenty of time for meals
   - Be prepared to adapt to changing needs or preferences
6. **Create a calm environment:**
   - Speak in a gentle, encouraging tone
   - Play soft background music if it's soothing
7. **Use visual and aromatic cues:**
   - Let your loved one see and smell the food being prepared
   - Use descriptive language to stimulate appetite

Everyone is unique; what works one day may not work the next. Be prepared to adapt and stay positive.

Planning and preparing meals for someone with dementia requires creativity, patience, and flexibility. Focusing on nutrition, adapting familiar recipes, and creating a positive atmosphere can make mealtimes more enjoyable and nourishing for your loved one.

Remember to take care of yourself too. Meal preparation can be time-consuming, so don't hesitate to ask for help or use convenience foods when needed. Your well-being is crucial in providing the best care for your loved one.

Your efforts in providing nutritious, enjoyable meals are a profound expression of care and love. Even on challenging days, know that dedication significantly affects your loved one's quality of life.

When to Seek Professional Help

As a caregiver or family member of someone with dementia, it's crucial to recognize when professional help is needed for nutritional concerns. Your attentiveness and quick action can significantly impact your loved one's health and quality of life. Let's explore the signs that indicate a need for medical or nutritional intervention and how to work effectively with healthcare providers.

Signs that Indicate the Need for Medical or Nutritional Intervention

It's essential to be vigilant and watch for these key indicators that suggest your loved one may need professional help:

1. **Significant Weight Changes:**
   - Unexplained weight loss of 5% or more in a month
   - Rapid weight gain that may indicate fluid retention
2. **Eating Behaviors:**
   - Consistently refusing meals
   - Difficulty chewing or swallowing
   - Frequent choking or coughing while eating
3. **Physical Signs:**
   - Dry, cracked lips or mouth sores
   - Sunken eyes or cheeks
   - Muscle wasting or weakness
4. **Digestive Issues:**
   - Frequent constipation or diarrhea
   - Persistent nausea or vomiting
5. **Cognitive and Behavioral Changes:**
   - Increased confusion or agitation around mealtimes
   - Forgetting how to use utensils
   - Holding food in the mouth without swallowing
6. **Skin Conditions:**
   - Slow wound healing
   - Development of pressure sores
7. **Hydration Concerns:**

- Dark, strong-smelling urine
- Decreased urine output
- Increased thirst

Red Flags for Nutritional Concerns in Dementia

Category	Warning Signs	Potential Implications
Weight	Sudden loss or gain	Malnutrition or fluid retention
Eating	Refusal, choking, difficulty swallowing	Dysphagia, aspiration risk
Physical	Dry mouth, muscle wasting	Dehydration, protein deficiency
Digestive	Constipation, diarrhea	Malabsorption, medication side effects
Cognitive	Increased confusion at mealtimes	Disease progression, medication issues
Skin	Slow healing, pressure sores	Protein/vitamin deficiency, immobility
Hydration	Dark urine, decreased output	Dehydration risk

Working with Healthcare Providers to Address Nutritional Concerns

When you notice these signs, it's time to collaborate with healthcare professionals. Here's how to effectively work with them:

1. **Prepare for the Appointment:**
   - Keep a detailed food and drink diary for at least a week
   - Note any changes in medication or routine
   - Write down specific concerns and questions
2. **Communicate Clearly:**
   - Be specific about the changes you've observed
   - Provide concrete examples and timelines
   - Don't hesitate to ask for clarification if you don't understand something
3. **Seek a Comprehensive Assessment:**
   - Request a complete nutritional evaluation
   - Ask about blood tests to check for vitamin deficiencies or other issues
   - Inquire about a swallowing assessment if relevant
4. **Discuss Treatment Options:**
   - Ask about dietary modifications
   - Explore the possibility of nutritional supplements
   - Inquire about medication adjustments if side effects are impacting nutrition

5. **Develop a Care Plan:**
   - Work with the healthcare team to create a personalized nutrition plan
   - Ensure the plan is realistic and manageable for your caregiving situation
   - Discuss how to monitor progress and when to follow up
6. **Seek Referrals if Needed:**
   - Ask about consulting a dietitian specializing in dementia care
   - Inquire about speech therapy for swallowing difficulties
   - Consider occupational therapy for assistance with eating skills
7. **Stay Informed and Proactive:**
   - Keep all healthcare providers informed of changes or new concerns
   - Don't wait for scheduled appointments if urgent issues arise
   - Participate in caregiver education programs offered by healthcare providers

Remember: You are essential to your loved one's healthcare team. Your observations and input are invaluable in ensuring they receive the best possible care.

Final Thoughts:

Recognizing when to seek professional help for nutritional concerns is a critical aspect of caregiving for someone with dementia. By staying alert to the signs and working closely with healthcare providers, you can help ensure your loved one maintains the best nutritional status and quality of life.

Don't hesitate to ask for help—healthcare professionals support you and your loved one. Your proactive approach to seeking assistance is a testament to your dedication and care. Remember, taking care of your loved one's nutritional needs is a team effort, and you play a crucial role in that team.

By staying informed, observant, and collaborative with healthcare providers, you're providing the best possible care for your loved one. Your efforts in this challenging journey are commendable and make a significant difference in their well-being.

Preparing for End-of-Life Decisions

While difficult to contemplate, preparing for end-of-life decisions is essential to caregiving. Having these conversations and making plans can provide peace of mind and ensure your loved one's wishes are respected.

Steps in Preparing for End-of-Life Decisions:

1. **Start the Conversation**
    - Choose a calm moment to discuss end-of-life wishes with your loved one.
    - Approach the topic with sensitivity and openness.

2. **Understand Your Loved One's Wishes**
    - Discuss preferences for medical interventions, pain management, and place of care.
    - Explore spiritual or cultural considerations.

3. **Document Decisions**
    - Ensure advance directives (living will, healthcare power of attorney) are in place.
    - Consider creating a POLST (Physician Orders for Life-Sustaining Treatment) form.

4. **Communicate with Healthcare Providers**
    - Share documented wishes with all relevant healthcare providers.
    - Ensure copies of advance directives are in medical records.

5. **Plan for Practical Matters**
    - Discuss funeral or memorial preferences.
    - Address financial and legal matters (wills, estate planning).

6. **Prepare Emotionally**
    - Seek support from counselors, support groups, or spiritual advisors.
    - Allow yourself to process emotions as you plan.

7. **Focus on Quality of Life**
    - Discuss what quality of life means to your loved one.
    - Align care decisions with these values.

End-of-Life Consideration	Questions to Discuss	Documentation Needed
Medical Interventions	Preferences for resuscitation, ventilation, feeding tubes	Living Will, POLST Form
Pain Management	Comfort goals, medication preferences	Advance Directive, Pain Management Plan
Place of Care	Preference for home, hospital, or hospice care	Documented in Advance Care Plan
Spiritual/Cultural Needs	Desired rituals, religious support	Noted in Personal Directive

Remember, coping with grief and loss is a profoundly personal journey. There's no right or wrong way to feel; seeking help is okay. By acknowledging your grief, finding meaning in your caregiving role, and preparing for difficult decisions, you're honoring both yourself and your loved one.

These conversations and preparations, while challenging, can bring a sense of peace and allow you to focus on creating meaningful moments with your loved one. Don't hesitate to lean on your support network, seek professional help if needed, and be gentle with yourself throughout this process. Your role as a caregiver is invaluable, and taking care of your emotional well-being is essential to providing compassionate care.

When to Consider Hospice

Hospice care is a compassionate approach to end-of-life care that focuses on comfort, quality of life, and dignity. It's important to understand that choosing hospice doesn't mean giving up – it means shifting the focus from curative treatment to comfort care.

Critical aspects of hospice care include:

1. Pain management and symptom control
2. Emotional and spiritual support for the patient and family
3. Assistance with personal care and daily living activities
4. Respite care for family caregivers
5. Bereavement support for loved ones

Hospice care is typically provided by a team of professionals, including:

- Doctors
- Nurses
- Social workers
- Chaplains or spiritual advisors
- Trained volunteers

Hospice Service	Description
Medical Care	Pain management, symptom control, and medication management.
Personal Care	Assistance with bathing, dressing, and other daily activities.
Emotional Support	Counseling for patient and family, addressing fears and concerns.
Spiritual Care	Support for spiritual needs and end-of-life rituals.
Practical Support	Help with household tasks, errands, and respite care.

The importance of timely hospice involvement

Deciding when to involve hospice care can be emotionally challenging, but **early involvement often leads to better outcomes** for both the person with dementia and their caregivers. Here's why timely hospice care is crucial:

1. **Improved quality of life**: Hospice teams are experts in managing pain and other symptoms, helping your loved one feel more comfortable.

2. **Reduced hospitalizations**: Proper symptom management often reduces the need for emergency room visits or hospital stays.

3. **Emotional and spiritual support**: Hospice offers counseling and support services that benefit you and your loved one.

4. **Time to say goodbye**: Earlier involvement gives family members more time to spend with their loved one and address unfinished business.

5. **Caregiver support**: Hospice provides education, resources, and respite care to help you navigate this challenging time.

Remember, choosing hospice doesn't mean death is imminent. Many patients receive hospice care for months, allowing them to make the most of their remaining time with improved comfort and quality of life.

Benefits of Early Hospice Involvement	Impact on Patient and Family
Better symptom management	Increased comfort and reduced suffering
Comprehensive support	Improved overall quality of life for the patient and caregivers
Avoid crises	Less stress and anxiety for family members
Time for meaningful moments	Opportunity to create lasting memories and say goodbyes

By understanding dementia, hospice care, and the benefits of timely involvement, you're better equipped to make informed decisions about your loved one's care. Remember, you're not alone in this journey – hospice teams are there to support both you and your loved one every step of the way.

Signs It May Be Time for Hospice Care

As a caregiver or family member of someone with dementia, recognizing when it's time to consider hospice care can be challenging. This decision is deeply personal and often emotional. However, certain signs can help guide you in making this vital choice. Let's explore these indicators in detail.

Physical indicators

Physical changes are often the most noticeable signs that your loved one's condition is progressing. **Look for these physical indicators**:

1. **Significant weight loss**: A 10% or more decrease in body weight in six months.

2. **Frequent infections**: Pneumonia or urinary tract infections that are becoming harder to treat.

3. **Difficulty swallowing**: This can lead to choking, coughing during meals, or refusal to eat.

4. **Increased pain**: Despite efforts to manage it with medication.

5. **Skin breakdown**: Pressure sores or other skin issues that aren't healing.

6. **Changes in breathing**: Shortness of breath, labored breathing, or long pauses between breaths.

7. **Decreased mobility**: Becoming bed-bound or unable to sit up without support.

Physical Indicator	What to Look For
Weight Loss	Loose clothing, visible bone structure, sunken cheeks
Swallowing Difficulties	Coughing during meals, holding food in the mouth, refusing to eat
Skin Issues	Redness, open sores, slow healing of wounds
Mobility Changes	Inability to walk independently, frequent falls, reluctance to move

Cognitive and behavioral changes

As dementia progresses, you may notice significant changes in your loved one's cognitive abilities and behavior. **Fundamental changes to watch for include**:

- Increased confusion and disorientation
- Difficulty recognizing family members
- Loss of ability to communicate verbally
- Agitation, aggression, or combative behavior
- Withdrawal from social interactions
- Changes in sleep patterns (sleeping more during the day, restless at night)
- Hallucinations or delusions

Remember, these changes can be distressing for you and your loved one. Hospice care can help you manage these symptoms and improve your quality of life.

Frequent hospitalizations or ER visits

If you find yourself taking your loved one to the emergency room or hospital more often, it might be time to consider hospice care. **Signs to consider include**:

1. Multiple hospitalizations within the past six months
2. Recurring infections or illnesses
3. Increasing difficulty managing symptoms at home
4. Longer recovery times after each hospital stay

Frequency of Medical Visits	Consideration
1-2 ER visits in 6 months	Monitor closely and consult with a doctor.
3+ ER visits in 6 months	This is a strong indication for a hospice evaluation.
Any hospital stay longer than one week	Consider hospice discussion.

Decline in daily functioning

A significant decline in your loved one's ability to perform daily tasks independently is a strong indicator that hospice care may be beneficial. **Watch for**:

- Inability to dress, bathe, or groom without assistance
- Incontinence or loss of bladder and bowel control
- Difficulty moving from bed to chair without help
- Inability to prepare or eat meals independently
- Decreased interest in previously enjoyed activities

These changes often mean that your loved one requires more intensive care, which hospice can provide while ensuring comfort and dignity.

In conclusion, deciding when to consider hospice care is complex and personal. By being aware of these signs – physical changes, cognitive decline, frequent hospitalizations, and decreased daily functioning – you can make a more informed choice about when to seek additional support. Remember, hospice care is not about giving up hope; it's about ensuring the best possible quality of life for your loved one and support for you as a caregiver.

The Benefits of Hospice Care for Dementia Patients

When considering hospice care for your loved one with dementia, it's essential to understand the numerous benefits this specialized care can provide. Hospice focuses on comfort and quality of life, offering a holistic approach to supporting the patient and their family. Let's explore these benefits in detail.

Pain management and symptom control

One of the primary goals of hospice care is to ensure that your loved one is as comfortable as possible. **Effective pain management and symptom control can significantly improve their quality of life.**

Critical aspects of pain and symptom management in hospice care include:

1. **Personalized pain assessment**: Hospice professionals are trained to recognize pain in patients who cannot communicate verbally.

2. **Tailored medication plans**: Medications are carefully selected and adjusted to provide maximum comfort with minimal side effects.

3. **Non-pharmacological interventions** may include massage, music therapy, or aromatherapy to complement medication.

4. **Regular monitoring**: The hospice team assesses the patient's comfort level and adjusts care as needed.

5. **Management of other symptoms**: This includes addressing issues like shortness of breath, nausea, anxiety, and sleep disturbances.

Common Dementia Symptoms	Hospice Management Approach
Pain	Tailored pain medication, positioning, gentle massage
Agitation	Calming techniques, environmental adjustments, medication if necessary
Difficulty swallowing	Dietary modifications, proper positioning, oral care
Skin issues	Regular repositioning, specialized mattresses, wound care

Emotional and spiritual support

Hospice care recognizes that emotional and spiritual well-being is as important as physical comfort. **This holistic approach can provide immense comfort to the patient and their family.**

Emotional and spiritual support in hospice care includes:

- Counseling services for the patient and family members
- Support from social workers to address practical and emotional concerns
- Chaplain services for spiritual support, regardless of religious affiliation
- Assistance with life review and legacy projects
- Grief counseling for family members, both before and after their loved one's passing

Remember, this support is tailored to your family's needs and beliefs. The hospice team is there to provide comfort and guidance, not to impose any particular spiritual or religious views.

Respite care for family caregivers

Caring for a loved one with dementia can be physically and emotionally exhausting. **Hospice care recognizes the vital role of family caregivers and offers respite services to prevent burnout.**

Respite care benefits include:

1. Short-term relief from caregiving duties
2. Opportunity for self-care and rest
3. Time to attend to personal matters or other family responsibilities
4. Professional care for your loved one, ensuring their needs are met
5. Reduced stress and improved overall well-being for the caregiver

Improved quality of life

The ultimate goal of hospice care is to improve the patient's and their family's overall quality of life. **This is achieved through expert care, support, and a focus on comfort rather than curative treatments.**

Ways hospice care can improve quality of life:

- Allowing the patient to remain in familiar surroundings, often at home
- Providing equipment and supplies necessary for comfort and care
- Offering 24/7 support and guidance for family caregivers
- Facilitating meaningful interactions and moments between the patient and their loved ones
- Ensuring dignity and respect in all aspects of care

Addressing not just physical needs but also emotional, social, and spiritual needs Quality of Life Aspect	Hospice Care Impact
Comfort	Reduced pain and distressing symptoms.
Dignity	Personalized care respecting individual preferences.
Family connection	Support for meaningful interactions and memory-making.
Peace of mind	24/7 professional support and guidance.

In conclusion, hospice care offers numerous benefits for dementia patients and their families. By focusing on comprehensive symptom management, providing emotional and spiritual support, offering respite care, and striving to improve overall quality of life, hospice care can make a significant difference in your loved one's final months or years.

Remember, choosing hospice care doesn't mean giving up hope. Instead, it means shifting the focus to ensuring the best possible quality of life and comfort for your loved one. It's about making the most of your time together, creating meaningful moments, and finding peace in knowing your loved one receives expert, compassionate care.

Common Misconceptions About Hospice Care

When considering hospice care for a loved one with dementia, you may encounter several misconceptions that can cause hesitation or concern. Understanding the realities of hospice care is essential to making an informed decision. Let's address the most common misconceptions and clarify what hospice care entails.

Hospice is not giving up.

One of the most pervasive misconceptions about hospice care is that it means "giving up" on your loved one. **This couldn't be further from the truth.**

Here's why hospice is not giving up:

1. **Shift in focus**: Hospice represents a change in care goals, not an abandonment of care. The focus shifts from curative treatments to comfort and quality of life.

2. **Active care**: Hospice provides expert care to manage symptoms and improve comfort.

3. **A holistic approach** addresses not just physical needs but also emotional, social, and spiritual aspects of well-being.

4. **Empowerment**: Hospice empowers patients and families to make choices about their care and how they want to spend their remaining time.

5. **Celebration of life**: Many hospice programs encourage life reviews and legacy projects, which celebrate the person's life and accomplishments.

Misconception	Reality
Hospice means no more treatment.	Hospice provides active treatment for symptoms and comfort.
Choosing hospice means giving up hope.	Hospice shifts hope to quality of life and meaningful moments.
Hospice is only for the last few days of life.	Hospice can provide care for months, enhancing life quality.

Hospice doesn't mean imminent death.

Another common misconception is that hospice care is only for the last few days or weeks of life. **Hospice care can be beneficial for months and sometimes even longer.**

Key points to understand:

- Hospice eligibility typically requires a prognosis of six months or less, but this is not a strict limit.

- Many patients receive hospice care for several months, with some even "graduating" from hospice if their condition stabilizes.

- Earlier involvement of hospice often leads to a better quality of life and can sometimes even extend life by reducing stress on the body.

- Hospice care can be discontinued if the patient's condition improves or if they decide to pursue curative treatments again.

Time in Hospice	Potential Benefits
Days to weeks	Immediate comfort care and family support in crisis
Weeks to months	Sustained symptom management, quality time with family
Months or longer	Long-term comfort, potential for stabilization or improvement

Hospice care can be provided at home.

Many people believe that choosing hospice care means their loved one must move to a facility. **Hospice care is often provided right in the comfort of the patient's home.**

Understanding home hospice care:

1. **Flexibility**: Hospice care can be provided wherever the patient calls home – private residences, assisted living facilities, or nursing homes.

2. **Customized care**: The hospice team works with you to create a care plan that fits your home environment and family dynamics.

3. **Equipment and supplies**: Necessary medical equipment (like hospital beds or oxygen) is provided and set up in the home.

4. **24/7 support**: While the hospice team isn't present 24/7, they're always available by phone for guidance and can visit as needed.

5. **Family involvement**: Home hospice allows family members to be intimately involved in care, with guidance from the hospice team.

6. **Familiar surroundings**: Patients often find comfort surrounded by familiar sights, sounds, and loved ones.

Aspect of Care	In-Home Hospice Provision
Medical care	Regular visits from nurses and doctors
Personal care	Assistance with bathing and dressing by hospice aides
Emotional support	Visits from social workers and counselors
Spiritual care	Chaplain visits if desired

It's important to note that while home hospice is common, inpatient hospice facilities are available for those who need or prefer that option. Some patients may transition between home and inpatient care as their needs change.

In conclusion, understanding these common misconceptions about hospice care can help you make a more informed decision for your loved one with dementia. Hospice is not about giving up or waiting for death; it's about living life as fully and comfortably as possible in whatever time remains. It offers expert care that can often be provided at home, surrounding your loved one with familiar comforts and loving family members.

Remember, choosing hospice care is a profoundly personal decision. It's okay to have questions and concerns. Don't hesitate to contact hospice providers in your area to learn more about their services and how they might benefit your loved one and your family. Your choice to consider hospice care demonstrates your commitment to ensuring the best possible quality of life for your loved one, which is an act of profound love and care.

How to Initiate the Hospice Conversation

Initiating a conversation about hospice care can be challenging and emotionally charged. However, having these discussions early can lead to better care decisions and more time to prepare. Here's how to approach this sensitive topic with compassion and clarity.

Talking with your loved one

When possible, it's essential to involve your loved one with dementia in the decision-making process. While their ability to participate may vary, including them shows respect for their wishes and autonomy.

Tips for talking with your loved one:

1. **Choose the right time and place**: Find a quiet, comfortable setting where your loved one is most alert and receptive.

2. **Be direct but gentle**: Use clear, simple language. Avoid euphemisms that might confuse them.

3. **Listen actively**: Pay attention to their verbal and non-verbal responses.

4. **Respect their feelings**: Acknowledge any fears or concerns they express.

5. **Focus on the benefits**: Explain how hospice can help manage their symptoms and improve comfort.

6. **Be patient.** This may need to be an ongoing conversation. Don't rush to decide everything in one sitting.

Use visual aids: If appropriate, consider using brochures or videos to help explain hospice care. **What to Say**	**What to Avoid**
"I want to talk about how we can keep you comfortable."	"We need to discuss end-of-life care."
"Hospice can help us manage your pain better."	"There's nothing more we can do for you."
"What's most important to you right now?"	"You should consider hospice care."

Discussing with family members

Bringing up hospice care with other family members can sometimes be as challenging as discussing it with your loved one. Family dynamics, differing opinions, and emotional responses can complicate these conversations.

Strategies for family discussions:

- **Plan**: Consider who should be part of the conversation and how to involve distant family members.

- **Choose a spokesperson**: Designate one person to lead the conversation if helpful.

- **Share information**: Before the discussion, provide educational materials about hospice care to all family members.

- **Be inclusive**: Ensure everyone has a chance to express their thoughts and feelings.

- **Focus on your loved one's wishes**: If known, center the discussion on what your loved one with dementia would want.

- **Address concerns**: Be open to questions and address fears or misconceptions about hospice care.

Seek professional help: Consider involving a social worker or counselor to facilitate the conversation if family conflicts arise.	Possible Responses
Common Family Concerns	
"Isn't this giving up?"	"Hospice focuses on quality of life and comfort, not giving up."
"It's too soon to consider hospice."	"Earlier hospice involvement often leads to better care and support."
"We can't afford it."	"Medicare, Medicaid, and most private insurances usually cover hospice."

Consulting with healthcare providers

Healthcare providers play a crucial role in the decision to pursue hospice care. They can provide valuable insights into your loved one's condition and prognosis and help you understand if hospice is appropriate.

Steps for consulting healthcare providers:

1. **Schedule a dedicated appointment**: Request a meeting to discuss your loved one's care options, including hospice.

2. **Prepare questions**: Write down your questions and concerns beforehand. Some key questions might include:
   - Is my loved one eligible for hospice care?
   - How might hospice benefit them at this stage?
   - What changes in their condition should we be watching for?

3. **Bring support**: Consider having another family member present to help remember information.

4. **Take notes**: Write down important points or ask if you can record the conversation for future reference.

5. **Discuss prognosis**: While difficult, understanding the expected progression of your loved one's condition can help you make decisions.

6. **Ask about referrals**: If hospice seems appropriate, ask for referrals to reputable hospice providers in your area.

7. **Follow-up**: Don't hesitate to contact the healthcare provider with any additional questions after the meeting.

Healthcare Provider	Role in Hospice Discussion
Primary Care Physician	Overall health assessment and long-term care planning.
Neurologist	Dementia progression and symptom management.
Geriatrician	Specialized care needs for older adults.
Palliative Care Specialist	Expert in comfort care and quality of life issues.

Remember, initiating the hospice conversation is an act of love and care. It shows that you're thinking proactively about ensuring the best possible quality of life for your loved one. While these discussions can be difficult, they often bring a sense of relief and clarity once they're underway.

It's normal to feel a range of emotions during this process. Don't hesitate to seek support for yourself, whether from friends, support groups, or professional counselors. Taking care of your emotional well-being is crucial as you navigate this challenging journey.

Ultimately, the goal is to make informed decisions that honor your loved one's wishes and provide them with the most appropriate and compassionate care possible. By approaching these conversations with openness, empathy, and a focus on your loved one's well-being, you can navigate this critical decision-making process with greater confidence and peace of mind.

The Hospice Evaluation Process

Understanding the hospice evaluation process can help alleviate some of the anxiety and uncertainty you may feel when considering this option for your loved one with dementia. This process ensures that hospice care is appropriate and tailored to your loved one's specific needs. Let's explore each step in detail.

Eligibility criteria for dementia patients

Specific criteria apply to people with dementia who are eligible for hospice care. **These criteria are guidelines, and each case is evaluated individually.**

Key eligibility factors for dementia patients include:

1. **Disease progression**: The person should be in the late stages of dementia, typically stage 7, on the Functional Assessment Staging Test (FAST).

2. **Functional decline**: Inability to perform daily activities without substantial assistance.

3. **Medical complications**: Presence of conditions such as aspiration pneumonia, upper urinary tract infections, sepsis, or multiple stage 3-4 pressure ulcers.

4. **Nutritional decline**: Difficulty eating and swallowing, leading to weight loss.

5. **Verbal communication**: Limited to fewer than six intelligible daily words.

6. **Mobility**: Unable to walk without assistance and eventually becoming bed-bound.

Eligibility Factor	Description
FAST Stage 7	Very severe cognitive decline, minimal verbal communication
ADL Dependence	Requires help with most or all activities of daily living
Medical Complications	Recurrent infections, difficulty swallowing, pressure sores
Nutritional Decline	Significant weight loss, difficulty eating independently

Remember, meeting these criteria doesn't automatically mean hospice is the right choice, nor does failing to meet all requirements necessarily disqualify someone. The decision involves a comprehensive evaluation by healthcare professionals and discussions with the family.

What to expect during the evaluation

The hospice evaluation is a thorough process designed to assess your loved one's needs and determine whether hospice care is appropriate. **It is typically provided at no cost and does not obligate you to choose hospice care**.

The evaluation process usually includes:

- **Initial consultation**: A hospice representative will meet with you and your loved one to explain services and answer questions.
- **Medical review**: The hospice team will review your loved one's medical history and condition.
- **Physical assessment**: A nurse will conduct a physical examination to evaluate symptoms and care needs.
- **Psychosocial assessment**: A social worker may assess emotional needs and family dynamics.
- **Home safety evaluation**: If care will be provided at home, the team will assess the environment for safety and equipment needs.
- **Discussion of goals**: The team will discuss your loved one's care goals and preferences with you.

Evaluation Step	Conducted By
Initial Consultation	Hospice Representative
Medical Review	Hospice Physician
Physical Assessment	Hospice Nurse
Psychosocial Assessment	Social Worker

Creating a care plan

If your loved one is found eligible for hospice and you decide to proceed, the next step is creating a personalized care plan. This plan is a **collaborative effort** between the hospice team, your loved one (if able to participate), and your family.

The care plan typically includes:

1. **Symptom management strategies**: Plans for managing pain, anxiety, breathing difficulties, and other symptoms.
2. **Medication regimen**: A review and adjustment of current medications, focusing on comfort and symptom control.
3. **Personal care routines**: Plans for bathing, feeding, and other daily care needs.
4. **Emotional and spiritual support**: Arrange counseling, chaplain visits, or other support services.
5. **Family education**: Training for family caregivers on providing care and recognizing important signs or symptoms.
6. **Emergency procedures**: Clear instructions on what to do in case of emergencies or sudden changes in condition.
7. **Respite care arrangements**: Plans for providing breaks to family caregivers.

Care Plan Component	Purpose
Symptom Management	Ensure comfort and quality of life.
Medication Management	Optimize effectiveness and minimize side effects.
Personal Care	Maintain dignity and prevent complications.
Emotional Support	Address the psychological needs of the patient and family.

It's important to understand that the care plan is a **dynamic document**. It will be regularly reviewed and adjusted as your loved one's needs change. You and your family will be integral parts of this ongoing process.

Remember, the hospice evaluation and care planning process ensures your loved one receives the most appropriate and compassionate care possible. It's an opportunity to ask questions, express concerns, and actively participate in shaping your loved one's care.

Don't hesitate to ask for clarification if anything is unclear during this process. The hospice team supports you and your loved one every step of the way. They aim to honor your loved one's wishes, provide expert care, and help your entire family through this challenging time.

By understanding and actively participating in the evaluation and care planning process, you're taking an essential step in ensuring the best possible care and quality of life for your loved one with dementia. While sometimes emotional, this process can also bring relief and clarity as you navigate this difficult journey.

Preparing for Hospice Care

Once you've decided to pursue hospice care for your loved one with dementia, there are several important steps to take to ensure a smooth transition. This preparation phase is crucial for creating a supportive environment and understanding what to expect. Let's explore these steps in detail.

Choosing a Hospice Provider

Selecting the right hospice provider is a critical decision that can significantly impact the quality of care your loved one receives. **Take your time with this process, and don't hesitate to ask questions.**

Consider the following when choosing a hospice provider:

1. **Certification and accreditation**: Ensure the provider is Medicare-certified and, ideally, accredited by a national organization.
2. **Range of services**: Look for providers offering comprehensive medical, emotional, and spiritual support.
3. **Availability**: Choose a provider that offers 24/7 emergency on-call services.

4. **Experience with dementia**: Ask about their specific experience in caring for patients with dementia.

5. **Staff qualifications**: Inquire about the training and qualifications of their care team members.

6. **Respite care options**: Check if they offer respite care to give family caregivers breaks.

7. **Bereavement support**: Look for providers that offer grief counseling and support after your loved one's passing.

Question to Ask	Why It's Important
How quickly can you start services?	Ensures timely care initiation
What is your staff-to-patient ratio?	Indicates the level of individual attention
How do you manage pain in dementia patients?	Reveals expertise in dementia-specific care
What support do you offer family caregivers?	Indicates the level of family involvement and support

Setting up the care environment

Creating a safe, comfortable environment is essential for hospice care, especially if your loved one will be cared for at home. **The goal is to promote comfort, safety, and ease of care.**

Critical considerations for setting up the care environment:

- **Bedroom setup**: Ensure the bed is accessible from both sides. If recommended by the hospice team, consider a hospital bed.

- **Bathroom modifications**: Install grab bars, a raised toilet seat, and non-slip mats if needed.

- **Clear pathways**: Remove clutter and ensure clear paths for easy movement, primarily if a wheelchair or walker is used.

- **Lighting**: Provide adequate lighting to prevent falls and aid in care tasks.

- **Comfortable seating**: Have a comfortable chair for your loved one and seating for visitors.
- **Temperature control**: Ensure the room can be kept at a comfortable temperature.
- **Meaningful objects**: Include photos, favorite blankets, or other cherished items to create a comforting atmosphere.

Item	Purpose
Hospital bed	Allows for positioning adjustments, easier care
Bedside commode	Reduces the need for bathroom trips
Over-bed table	Provides surface for meals, activities
Night light	Improves safety during nighttime care

Understanding your role as a caregiver

As a family caregiver, your role will evolve with the introduction of hospice care. **While the hospice team will provide expert care, your involvement remains crucial.**

Your role as a caregiver may include:

1. **Being an advocate**: You know your loved one best. Share insights about their preferences, behaviors, and needs with the hospice team.
2. **Providing comfort**: Your presence and touch can be incredibly comforting. Spend time with your loved one, hold their hand, or sit with them.
3. **Assisting with personal care**: The hospice team will guide you in helping with feeding, bathing, or repositioning.
4. **Medication management**: While the hospice team will manage medications, you may be involved in administering them.
5. **Emotional support**: Provide reassurance and emotional support to your loved one.
6. **Communication liaison**: Keep other family members informed about your loved one's condition and care.

7. **Self-care**: Remember to take care of yourself too. Accept help and take breaks when needed.

Caregiver Task	Hospice Team Support
Personal care assistance	Training on safe techniques, along with regular help from hospice aides
Medication administration	Clear instructions, regular check-ins, 24/7 phone support
Emotional support	Counseling services, tips for communication
Recognizing changes in condition	Education on what to watch for, when to call for help

Remember, the hospice team supports you and your loved one. **Don't hesitate to ask for help or clarification when you need it.** They can provide training, answer questions, and support you as you navigate this new role.

Preparing for hospice care can feel overwhelming, but taking these steps can help create a smoother transition. By choosing the right provider, setting up a comfortable environment, and understanding your role, you're laying the groundwork for compassionate, quality care for your loved one.

This preparation phase is also a time for emotional readiness. It's normal to feel a mix of emotions – relief, sadness, anxiety, or even guilt. Remember that choosing hospice care is an act of love, focusing on comfort and quality of life for your loved one. Don't hesitate to lean on the hospice team, friends, or support groups for emotional support.

By taking these steps to prepare, you're ensuring that your loved one will receive the best possible care in their final stage of life while also setting yourself up to be an informed and supported caregiver. Your dedication to this process is a testament to your love and commitment to your family member's well-being.

Navigating the Emotional Journey

The decision to pursue hospice care for a loved one with dementia marks the beginning of a profound emotional journey. This period can be filled with complex feelings and challenges. Understanding these emotions and finding coping methods is crucial for you and your loved one. Let's explore this journey and discuss strategies for navigating it with resilience and grace.

Coping with grief and anticipatory loss

Grief is a natural response to loss, and it often begins well before the actual passing of a loved one. This is known as anticipatory grief. **Recognizing and acknowledging these feelings is an essential step in coping with them.**

Common experiences of anticipatory grief include:

- Sadness and tearfulness
- Anxiety about the future
- Anger or frustration
- Guilt over past events or current feelings
- A sense of helplessness
- Difficulty concentrating
- Physical symptoms like fatigue or changes in appetite

Strategies for coping with anticipatory grief:

1. **Acknowledge your feelings**: Allow yourself to feel whatever emotions arise without judgment.
2. **Share your feelings**: Talk to trusted friends, family members, or a professional counselor.
3. **Practice self-compassion**: Be kind to yourself. Grief is a normal and valid response to your situation.
4. **Stay connected**: Maintain relationships with friends and family. Don't isolate yourself.
5. **Take care of your physical health**: Eat well, exercise, and get enough sleep.
6. **Find healthy outlets**: Engage in activities that help you process your emotions, such as journaling, art, or music.

7. **Stay present**: While worrying about the future is natural, focus on the present moment and your time with your loved one.

Grief Response	Coping Strategy
Overwhelming sadness	Allow yourself to cry; talk to a supportive friend.
Anxiety about the future	Practice mindfulness; focus on one day at a time.
Guilt over negative feelings	Practice self-compassion; join a support group.
Physical exhaustion	Prioritize self-care; ask for help with tasks.

Finding support for caregivers

Caring for a loved one with dementia in hospice care can be emotionally and physically demanding. **Seeking support is not a sign of weakness but a necessary step in maintaining your well-being.**

Options for caregiver support include:

- **Support groups**: Join groups specifically for dementia caregivers or hospice families. These can be in-person or online.

- **Professional counseling**: Consider individual therapy to process emotions and develop coping strategies.

- **Respite care**: Take your hospice provider's respite services for necessary breaks.

- **Family and friends**: Don't hesitate to ask for and accept help from your support network.

- **Educational resources**: Attend workshops or webinars about caregiving and end-of-life care to feel more prepared.

- **Spiritual or religious support**: If applicable, seek guidance from spiritual leaders or faith communities.

- **Self-care activities**: Engage in activities that recharge you, even for short periods.

Type of Support	Benefits
Caregiver support groups	Shared experiences, practical tips, emotional validation.
Professional counseling	Personalized coping strategies and safe space to process emotions.
Respite care	Time for self-care and reduced burnout risk.
Educational resources	Increased confidence in caregiving, better preparedness.

Celebrating life and creating meaningful moments

While this time is undoubtedly challenging, it also presents opportunities to celebrate your loved one's life and create lasting memories. **Focusing on positive experiences can provide comfort and meaning during this challenging journey.**

Ideas for creating meaningful moments:

1. **Life review**: Remember happy memories, perhaps creating a scrapbook or memory box together.

2. **Music therapy**: Play your loved one's favorite songs or hymns. Music can often evoke positive responses, even in late-stage dementia.

3. **Sensory experiences**: Engage the senses with familiar scents, textures, or flavors that bring comfort.

4. **Nature connection**: If possible, spend time outdoors or bring nature inside with flowers or plants.

5. **Gentle touch**: Hold hands, give a soft massage, or sit close to provide comfort through touch.

6. **Family gatherings**: Organize small, quiet gatherings of close family and friends to share stories and love.

7. **Legacy projects**: Create something together that can be shared with future generations, like a recipe book or family tree.

8. **Spiritual practices**: If prayer, meditation, or other spiritual practices are essential to your loved one, engage in them.

Meaningful Activity	Potential Benefits
Looking at old photos	Stimulates memories and encourages storytelling.
Listening to favorite music	It evokes emotions and may improve mood.
Gentle hand massage	It provides comfort and promotes relaxation.
Reading aloud familiar stories	Offers comfort and maintains connection.

Remember, the goal is not to create grand gestures but to find moments of connection, comfort, and joy, however small they seem.

Navigating the emotional journey of hospice care for a loved one with dementia is undoubtedly challenging. It's a path filled with complex emotions, difficult decisions, and profound moments of love and connection. You can find strength and moments of peace by acknowledging your feelings, seeking support, and focusing on creating meaningful experiences.

It's important to remember that there's no "right" way to feel or grieve. Your journey is unique, and having good and bad days is okay. Be patient and compassionate with yourself as you navigate this path.

Lastly, don't forget that the hospice team supports you and your loved one. They can provide resources, counseling, and guidance to help you through this emotional journey. You're not alone in this process; reaching out for help when needed is a sign of strength and love for yourself and your loved one.

Legal and Financial Considerations

When caring for a loved one with dementia who is entering hospice care, it's important to consider legal and financial matters. These can be challenging topics, but planning can bring peace of mind and help avoid problems later. Let's look at some key things to consider.

Advance Directives and Power of Attorney

Advance directives say what kind of medical care your loved one wants if they can't speak for themselves. There are two main types:

1. Living Will. This document states what medical treatments your loved one wants or doesn't want at the end of life.

2. Healthcare Power of Attorney: This names someone to make medical decisions if your loved one can't.

Power of attorney is also crucial for money matters. It lets someone manage your loved one's finances if they can't do it themselves.

Why these papers matter:

- They make sure your loved one's wishes are followed
- They can prevent family arguments about care decisions
- They make it easier to handle bills and other money matters

Setting these up early is best while your loved one can still make decisions. If you haven't done this yet, talk to a lawyer who knows about elder law as soon as possible.

Document	What It Does
Living Will	States end-of-life care wishes
Healthcare Power of Attorney	Names someone to make medical decisions
Financial Power of Attorney	Names someone to handle money matters

Understanding Hospice Coverage and Costs

The good news is that Medicare, Medicaid, and most private insurance plans usually cover hospice care. This coverage includes:

- Doctor and nursing services
- Medical equipment and supplies
- Medications for symptom control and pain relief
- Short-term inpatient care, if needed
- Grief counseling for the patient and family

What's not covered:

- Room and board if the patient is at home or in a nursing facility
- Treatments aimed at curing the illness (instead of comfort care); such treatments can invalidate hospice services.

It's good to check with your hospice provider and insurance company to understand what's covered and what you might need to pay for.

Usually Covered	Usually Not Covered
Hospice team visits	Curative treatments (which can invalidate hospice services)
Medical equipment	Room and board at home
Medications for comfort	Care from providers outside the hospice

Additional Resources and Support Programs

Besides insurance, other programs might help with costs or provide extra support:

1. Veterans Benefits: If your loved one served in the military, they might qualify for special hospice benefits through the VA.
2. Social Security: Your loved one might be eligible for disability benefits if they're under 65.
3. Local Senior Services: Many communities have programs that offer seniors meals, transportation, or other help.
4. Alzheimer's Association: They offer support groups and education and can help you find local resources.
5. Area Agency on Aging: This government program can connect you with services in your area.

Don't be afraid to ask for help. Social workers at the hospice or your local senior center can often recommend programs that might help.

Resource	What It Offers
Veterans Benefits	Special hospice care for veterans
Social Security	Possible disability benefits
Alzheimer's Association	Support groups and education

Remember, dealing with legal and money matters can feel overwhelming, but it's integral to caring for your loved one. Don't hesitate to ask for help from professionals like lawyers, financial advisors, or social workers. They can guide you through these complex issues and help you make the best decisions for your family.

Conclusion

As we reach the end of this guide on nutrition and dementia care, it's essential to take a moment to reflect on the incredible journey you're undertaking as a caregiver. Your path is not easy, but it's filled with opportunities for love, compassion, and meaningful connection.

Throughout this book, we've explored the complex relationship between nutrition and dementia, from understanding the basics of brain-healthy foods to navigating the challenges of late-stage feeding. But beyond the practical advice and scientific information, we've uncovered a more profound truth: mealtime is about much more than just food.

In caring for a loved one with dementia, you're not just providing sustenance for their body—you're nourishing their soul. Every carefully prepared meal, every patient spoonful, and every moment spent sitting together at the table is an act of love. It's saying, "I'm here for you, I care about you, and I'll support you through this journey."

Remember, there's no one-size-fits-all approach to dementia care. What works today might not work tomorrow, and that's okay. The key is to remain flexible, patient, and kind to your loved one and yourself. Don't be afraid to adapt, try new things, and seek help when needed.

As you move forward, remember that your well-being is just as important as that of your loved one. Take time to care for yourself, recharge, and find moments of joy in your day. Your strength and resilience are remarkable, and nurturing yourself to continue providing the best care possible is crucial.

Lastly, never underestimate the power of your presence. Even in the late stages of dementia, when words may fail, and meals become challenging, your loving presence is the most nourishing gift you can offer. A gentle touch, a warm smile, or simply sitting together in comfortable silence can be profoundly comforting.

You're doing important, meaningful work. On the difficult days, remember that your efforts matter immensely. You're making a difference in your loved one's life, one meal, one moment at a time.

As you continue this journey, may you find strength in knowing you're not alone. A community of caregivers, healthcare professionals, and supporters is ready to help you. Reach out, ask for help, and know that your dedication and love make a difference.

Thank you for being so committed to providing the best care for your loved one with dementia. Your compassion and dedication are truly inspiring. As you close this book, I hope you feel more empowered, informed, and supported in your caregiving journey. Remember, in nourishing your loved one, you're also nourishing the beautiful bond between you – and that's a truly precious gift.

Resources

Associations

Alzheimer's Association at https://www.alz.org/

Dementia Society of America at http://www.dementiasociety.org

National Institute on Aging at https://www.nia.nih.gov/

National Alliance for Caregiving at http://www.caregiving.org

Family Caregiver Alliance at http://www.caregiver.org

American Sleep Apnea Association at https://www.sleepapnea.org/

Author Bio

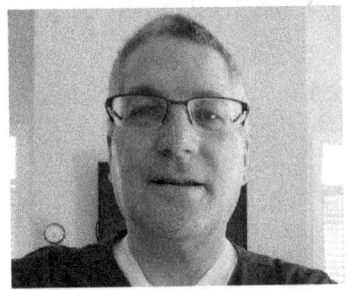 Peter Abraham, BSN, RN is an experienced nurse dedicated to supporting nurses, caregivers, families, and patients in their learning, growth, and well-being journey. Peter's nursing path encompasses practical experience as a cardiac telemetry nurse in a bustling cardiology unit at a Magnet-awarded teaching hospital. Additionally, Peter has fulfilled the role of a second-shift RN supervisor, overseeing an entire building in an SNF/LTC (Skilled Nursing Facility/Long-Term Care) setting with 151 residents. Remarkably, during the initial wave of COVID-19, the facility achieved an impressive close-to-100% recovery rate before operation warp speed was complete.

Furthermore, Peter's nursing career extends to rural home hospice care. As a visiting hospice registered nurse case manager, he offers compassionate care to patients in various settings, including private homes, personal care homes, assisted living facilities, skilled nursing facilities, and hospitals.

Moreover, Peter's desire to help others extends beyond his physical presence. At CompassionCrossing.Info, he writes articles to empower caregivers, family members, and fellow nurses in end-of-life care. Peter's drive to help others, which flows from his love of Christ Jesus, is a source of support and encouragement for all he reaches.

Other books by Peter Abraham include the following:

Empowering Excellence in Hospice: A Nurse's Toolkit for Best Practices series:

> Compliance-based, Eligibility Driven Hospice Documentation: Tips for Hospice Nurses
> Whispers of Time: Understanding the End-of-Life Timeline
> Terminal Clarity: Hospice Eligibility Guide for Nurses

Compassionate Caregiving series:

> Daily Hospice Care Planner: Organize, Communicate, and Provide Consistent Care
> Dignity in Dying: A Thoughtful Approach to Voluntary Stopping Eating and Drinking
> Palliative Sedation: A Compassionate Approach
> Hospice Medication Handbook: A Caregiver's Guide to Comfort Medications

Dementia Caregivers Essentials series:

> CPAP and Oxygen for Dementia
> Diabetes Care for Dementia
> Hallucination Management for Dementia
> Medication Compliance for Dementia
> Nutrition for Dementia
> Placement for Dementia
> Sundowning Management for Dementia

Connect with Peter On:

Website: https://compassioncrossing.info/